ARTHRITIS
ALTERNATIVES

ARTHRITIS ALTERNATIVES

IRNA AND LAURENCE GADD

Facts On File Publications
New York, New York ● Oxford, England

Library of Congress Cataloging in Publication Data

Gadd, Irna.
    Arthritis alternatives.

    Includes index.
    1. Arthritis.   2. Arthritis—Hospitals—Directories.
3. Arthritis—Societies, etc.—Directories.   4. Arthritis
—Information services—Directories.   I. Gadd, Laurence.
II. Title.
RC933.G33   1984   616.7'22   83-5642
ISBN 0-87196-769-3

                        Printed in the United States of America
                        10 9 8 7 6 5 4 3 2 1

ACKNOWLEDGMENTS

The editors wish to thank: the National Institute of Arthritis, Diabetes, and Digestive and Kidney Diseases for making available their fine research on rheumatic diseases; the many health professionals who took the time to participate in this effort; and John F. Thornton, the Associate Publisher at Facts On File, Inc., for his belief in the great need for the material in this volume.

In addition, for their interest and advice, we owe a debt of gratitude to Paul and Caren Goldberg, Neil and Carol Sherman, and Philip and Anne Roome. Above all, for their patience and understanding, we thank Alex and Emily.

CONTENTS

INTRODUCTION

This book serves a very specific purpose: the spreading of information. Lest that be taken as an obvious fact, please remember that, because of the overwhelming amount of information to be sifted and sorted through, people are too often happy to relinquish responsibility for their health care. The search for information may become a matter of going no further than to the nearest doctor (or to one who comes highly recommended by a friend or relative) for "the facts." The point is that facts go just so far; then judgment calls are needed. Rarely is there one unalterable "truth" when it comes to how to treat a disease or condition. In the case of arthritis, there are several different schools of thought regarding diagnosis and treatment. This book illustrates and illuminates them, in clear, jargon-free language.

One of the well-known elements in the successful treatment of any disease is the so-called placebo phenomenon: the patient will respond best to the treatment he or she believes in most. Increasingly today, people are aware that the traditional form of medicine practiced in the United States cannot always help people without causing side effects that often are as much of a problem as the original illness. It is known that other forms of treatment exist, but information concerning what they are and who practices them is not always readily available.

Throughout the book you will find the terms "traditional," "innovative," and "alternative" used to describe different approaches to the treatment of arthritis. Although many health professionals use two or even all three of these approaches in their treatment of arthritis, the distinction between the three can be generally defined as follows:

TRADITIONAL

Traditional medicine is often referred to as orthodox or allopathic medicine by those who practice other forms of treatment. It follows the course of diagnosis and treatment taught in U.S. medical and osteopathic schools, and is approved by the American Medical Association, The Arthritis Foundation, and the great majority of practicing physicians. Traditional treatment of arthritis relies extensively on drugs and, if thought necessary, surgery and physical therapy. Both Medical Doctors and Doctors of Osteopathy have similar training and, generally, their approaches to treatment are similar.

INNOVATIVE

The innovative approach to arthritis may be taken by a traditional medical doctor or an osteopath who uses a form of treatment he or she believes, based on formal research or empirical experience, to be more successful than the forms traditionally prescribed. In chapter six you will find many health professionals, hospitals, and clinics categorizing themselves as both traditional and innovative.

ALTERNATIVE

Generally, although many practitioners of alternative medicine are licensed medical doctors or osteopaths, the alternative approach to the treatment of arthritis is directly opposed to that of traditional medicine. The alternative practitioner usually uses minimal or non-invasive forms of treatment, avoiding drugs and surgery. Dietary supplements, vitamins, changes in diet, and acupuncture are some of the more common alternative approaches. Those health professionals who have classified themselves as alternative tend to be trained in homeopathy, chiropractic, naturopathy, bioecology, and nutrition.

The categories listed above have little or nothing to do with the actual training, degrees, or licenses of the particular health professional. They are indications of how the treatment of arthritis is currently approached by the individual practitioner. Remember that almost all treatment for arthritis is trial and error. It will take time, whatever approach your doctor uses, to find the specific treatment that will help you.

And so, back to the premise of this book. It is our hope that the information found herein will be of use to those who may want to consider other approaches to health care than those they have already tried and, perhaps, have found lacking. At very least, patients will have more information on the treatment they are receiving and, therefore, can be more active participants in their therapy. Also, with any condition as long-term as most rheumatic diseases are, treatment can reach what seems to be a dead end before the patient has achieved any real measure of recuperation. It may well be that the patient never will be rid completely of either the disease or its symptoms; even so, there are well-documented cases of people changing the mode of treatment and enjoying greater degrees of improvement.

It is not our purpose to advocate change for the sake of change, nor is it our place to advocate one form of treatment over another. Rather, we hope that by making the wide variety of treatments known, we will enable some of those who suffer from the various rheumatic diseases to make better informed choices and thereby recover a greater sense of well-being.

ARTHRITIS ALTERNATIVES

1

WHAT IS ARTHRITIS?

Arthritis. Say or read the words and most people think of aching joints, stiffness, and even crippling immobility. In truth, there is no one disease called "arthritis," and although the symptoms listed above certainly apply to some arthritic conditions, there are many other less well-known signs and symptoms than those three. These conditions can affect nearly every conceivable body structure, from joints to muscles, connective tissues, internal organs, and skin. The term rheumatic disease is used to describe the whole range of diseases most commonly referred to as arthritis and in layman's terms interchangeable.

Each arthritis patient, regardless of the form of the disease, will have his or her own particular set of symptoms of varying degree and duration. Some people have occasional flare-ups while others suffering from the same disease may be in constant discomfort. Many people have such slight symptoms that they are not even aware that they have arthritis; others are so severely affected that they can barely function. There is no way to know how any given patient will react to the progressive nature of arthritis or, in fact, to any particular treatment. Each case of arthritis is unique, and although it can be classified into one or more specific diseases, no predictions can be made as to its actual effect on any specific patient.

The word "arthritis" means inflammation of the joint. This is the best starting point for a discussion of arthritis, for it is just such inflammation and the resultant swelling and pain which most people associate with rheumatic disease.

The joints most often affected in arthritis are *synovial* joints, which are the mobile joints. These consist of the ends of two bones, each of which is coated with *cartilage*. Cartilage, a smooth tissue that enables the bone ends to move against each other easily, is sometimes called gristle by laymen. The entire joint is enclosed by a structure called the *capsule*, which is a continuation of the material that sheathes the bones. The capsule, in turn, is lined by the *synovial membrane* (also called the *synovium*). The synovium produces a fluid called *synovial fluid*, which functions to moisten the joint surfaces. Joints are acted upon by *ligaments*, which hold two bones together at the joint, and by *tendons*, which hold muscles to bones. These two structures are sometimes referred to as the *"soft tissues"* surrounding the joint.

Depending on which rheumatic condition a patient has, it may be the synovium that is affected initially, or the cartilage. But arthritis isn't limited to problems with synovial joints. Some arthritic disorders affect the entire body, including connective tissues and internal organs, and others affect the spine, or the skin (an organ in itself).

From this short capsulation, it is easy to understand why an arthritis sufferer cannot simply say "arthritis" and expect to get answers to questions about treatment. Other, more basic, questions must first be asked: Which particular form of the disease is manifest? How involved is it? What are the patient's major complaints? And these are just some of the questions that must be answered before treatment should be discussed.

CAUSES

Although arthritis is one of the earliest chronic diseases to have been recognized, and though more than 30 million Americans suffer from it, there is no clear answer to what causes the disease. More and more, research points out that various arthritic conditions can be detected by genetic markers, indicating heredity's role, yet not everyone with the markers develops the disease. Some doctors believe that all arthritic diseases are autoimmune conditions: The body is protected against disease by its immune mechanism, which attacks invading bacteria and other microorganisms. In an autoimmune disease, this mechanism becomes misdirected and works against the body itself. It is uncertain whether all of the varieties of rheumatic disease are autoimmune in nature, but systemic lupus erythematosus, for one, is considered to be so. Injury is sometimes thought to be the cause of rheumatic disease, but again, there is no hard evidence to support this theory. Often injury will bring on an arthritic condition, but not always. It might be that an injury can cause an already existing condition to become more noticeable. There are also some doctors and scientists who believe that infection is the primary trigger of arthritis. Some rheumatic diseases (Lyme arthritis, for one) result directly from infection and can be treated successfully if caught early enough.

Gout, now known to be one of the rheumatic diseases, was once thought to be a result of overindulgent eating. Some doctors today dispute diet as a cause of gout, whereas others maintain that not only gout, but all forms of arthritis, are at least affected by diet.

Some doctors would consider arthritis to be an allergy in every sense of the term, with certain foods being the allergens. This theory, too, is debated hotly in the medical profession.

It is clear that there is currently no universally accepted cause of arthritis. Furthermore, the traditional point of view is that until a cause can be identified, a cure will remain elusive. However, a large number of researchers and medical practitioners have claimed varying degrees of success in developing ways to control arthritis, even while lacking a sure knowledge of its cause, by carefully examining the empirical results to different forms of treatment.

THE DIFFERENT FORMS OF ARTHRITIS

What causes arthritis, how to cure it, how to prevent it—all these questions remain open to debate. What baffles the person seeking answers to these critical questions is that the various schools of treatment tend to dismiss the claims of the other schools. One thing the proponents of the various schools *do* agree on, however, is what characterizes each of the rheumatic conditions. The most common types are described below.

RHEUMATOID ARTHRITIS (often called Rheumatoid Disease) is one of the most common forms of arthritis. It can be crippling and deforming; it affects the synovium (therefore its designation as a form of synovitis) and the surrounding soft tissues of the joint; it can affect body organs if left untreated; and it affects women three times as often as men. Rheumatoid arthritis is not a disease of the old; it commonly affects people from 20 to 45 years of age.

The onset is slow and often unnoticeable as a form of arthritis because it can closely resemble a generalized virus. The first signs are usually muscle stiffness (particularly in the morning), tiredness, and aching and swelling of the joints, but weight loss and weakness may precede the awareness of real joint problems. Rheumatoid arthrithis affects joints unpredictably. It sometimes affects only the middle knuckles of the fingers or the hips and knees, but there does seem to be a symmetrical pattern to the disease. Both sides of the body tend to be affected in a "balanced" way. The degree of inflammation may be such that an individual is aware of discomfort only, or may be severe enought to be truly crippling.

As the disease progresses, the affected synovium is infiltrated by millions of cells which inflame and eventually thicken these otherwise thin membranes. The various parts of the joints are eaten away by collagenase, an enzyme that is activated by the inflammation. This erosion is the source of both the pain and crippling of rheumatoid arthritis. The crippling is a result of both the extreme damage to the synovium and the tightening of the muscles around the joint in response to the inflammation. Over time, prolonged tightening can cause the joint to dislocate and/or deform.

The problem of rheumatoid arthritis on a national scale is awesome: more than one million Americans suffer from it. The economic impact can be extreme, more because of inability to work than because of costliness of treatment.

OSTEOARTHRITIS (also known as osteoarthrosis) is often considered to be an inevitable part of old age. Although most cases are not diagnosed until the patient is advancing in years, some research shows that osteoarthritic-type changes can begin as early as the mid 20s. Osteo (a convenient, short form of the name) does not cripple the patient as a rule, and usually is not as painful as rheumatoid arthritis is. Those who do experience pain or stiffness find it to be an occasional problem, at worst. Osteo affects the cartilage that covers the bone ends in the joint; the cartilage literally wears away. In some cases the bone ends are exposed within the joint, and can become either pitted or thickened in response to the exposure. Osteo can ease with age if the exposed bone ends, in response to rubbing against each other, become smooth. This is called *eburnation*.

The most commonly known form of osteo, and also the mildest form, is that which affects the end joints of the fingers. The knobs at these joints are called *Heberden's nodes*, in commemoration of the doctor who first described them. In most cases, these knobs form slowly, and become visible in old age. The knarling of the finger joints and an occasional slight stiffness of the joints are the only symptoms of this type of osteo.

There are two other forms of osteo: one involves the spine, and the other the knees and hips. The spinal type is characterized by bony growths along the cervical (neck) or lower back vertebrae. In most cases there is an accompanying disintegration of the disks of the affected area. Surprisingly, there is little pain involved with this form of osteo; only when nerves are pinched or other pressure is applied to the nerves does the patient have pain. Often the condition is discovered by chance, when an x-ray of the back is taken for some other reason.

The third form of osteo, which involves weight-bearing joints, is potentially more serious. As noted above, the joints usually involved are the knees and hips, and both sides of the body are often affected. Pain can be severe enough to make walking difficult. Fluid frequently accumulates in the joint, often causing swelling. In extreme cases the knee is more severely affected on one side (i.e., inner or outer) than on the other, leading to bowing and even greater difficulty in walking and bearing weight.

GOUT is indeed a form of arthritis. At one time gout was associated with the rich, because it was thought to be caused by overindulgence in rich foods and drink. Modern research has shown that, while overindulgence can bring on an attack, the disease can affect anyone, although men are more frequent victims than women. Gout occurs when there is a buildup of uric acid crystals in the synovial fluid, with the knee and the big toe the most frequent targets. This buildup of crystals causes inflammation of the affected area.

There are two reasons for the buildup of the crystals; the first is that too much uric acid is produced in the body; the second is that the body cannot dispose of normal amounts of uric acid through the urine. Evidence for genetic tendency in gout is strong, yet an individual whose family has no history of the disease can be afflicted. Uric acid levels in the blood are also affected by stress and tension.

Although an elevated uric acid level is the underlying cause of gout, a person can go on for years with a higher-than-normal rate without developing the disease. Acute gouty arthritis begins when the uric acid level is so high that crystals begin to form and accumulate in the joint. When this happens, swelling occurs, the affected joint becomes red and tender, all in a period of a few hours. The attack will intensify, then peak in a few days. Typicallly, all symptoms of the incident ease gradually, and disappear after two weeks. Remarkably, after an attack has subsided, the joint and surrounding tissues appear to be normal.

Individuals who have endured an acute attack of gout still have elevated uric acid levels of the blood even after the attack, but crystallization does not occur constantly. There is another gouty condition which is chronic, called *chronic tophaceous gout.* Patients who suffer from it have such a high degree of crystallization that the crystals accumulate throughout the body in clumps called *tophi.* These deposits can be found almost anywhere, although they more commonly develop near joints, and sometimes occur directly under the skin near joints and in the ear. When the tophi develop within the bone near joints, the bone itself can be destroyed. The most dangerous place for tophi development is in the kidneys, because then kidney function is hampered.

PSEUDOGOUT, another form of arthritis, is similar to gout in many ways. In pseudogout, however, calcium pyrophosphate crystals, instead of uric acid crystals, are deposited in the synovium, and the crystals are formed in the cartilage rather than in the synovium. The accumulation of calcium in the cartilage appears to occur over a long period of time, with the pseudogout manifesting itself primarily in old age.

The symptoms of pseudogout resemble those of true gout, but attacks of the former tend to be less violent and, because the process of crystal depositing is more drawn-out, more protracted. One of the possible results of this disease is cartilage degeneration. When this occurs, the likelihood for prolonged active illness increases.

Some of the other differences between pseudogout and true gout are that, whereas gout affects men more than women, pseudogout seems impartial; pseudogout rarely involves the big toe, with the knee the most frequent site of attack; it is not unusual for several joints to be involved in pseudogout (wrists and ankles are often affected); and, as mentioned above, pseudogout appears to be a disease of old age, with the average age of first attack near 70.

JUVENILE RHEUMATOID ARTHRITIS is, as the name suggests, a disease of the young. The name is misleading, however, in that juvenile rheumatoid arthritis is not like rheumatoid arthritis in adults and, in fact, there really are three distinct types of the disease. Each has its own symptoms, and each has a different pattern of progression. They are: (1) systemic juvenile arthritis (also called Still's desease, or acute onset juvenile arthritis), poly-articular (meaning "many joints") juvenile arthritis, and monarti-cular (meaning "one joint") juvenile arthritis.

Systemic juvenile arthritis begins with a very high fever and a rash that seems to appear and disappear in concert with the fever. The patient generally feels sick, with muscle aches and exhaustion common. Equally typical is spleen, liver, and/or lymph node enlargement, but the joints will not necessarily be involved. The attack comes and goes abruptly, regardless of how long it lasts. It does recur, but there may be long intervals between attacks. Eventually joints will be affected with each attack, but that may take years to develop.

Polyarticular juvenile arthritis usually occurs with involvement of four or more joints, symmetrically distributed. Severe inflammation of the synovial membrane causes the joints to be tender, if not actually painful, swollen, and stiff. Symptoms also include listless-ness and sometimes weight loss. Typically, fever and rash occur only mildly, if at all, in this form.

The last kind of juvenile rheumatoid arthritis is called *monarticular juvenile arthritis*. Most often the knee is affected; if not the knee, the target is likely to be one of the larger joints. Aside from symptoms of the joint, few, if any, symptoms appear at all. The exception to this is in really young patients (younger than five, for example), who are likely to have such symptoms as fever, irritability, and general listlessness.

With juvenile rheumatoid arthritis, especially in the monarticular form, it is of the utmost importance to check with an ophthalmol-ogist regularly, for there can be eye involvement. The examination is, happily, a painless one, and if the eye condition (known as *chronic iridocyclitis*) is detected, it can be treated successfully.

Statistics indicate that more than half the children with JRA outgrow the disease; regrettably there is no way to predict which children will be the fortunate ones. The least likely to outgrow their diseases are those children who have the polyarticular form.

ACUTE RHEUMATIC FEVER, although a different disease from the three forms of juvenile rheumatoid arthritis, is included here because it can affect the joints (although it rarely damages them permanently) and, more seriously, can attack heart valves. This illness occurs after a streptococcal infection and, thanks to antibiotic treatment of strep throat, is now less common than in the past. Acute rheumatic fever actually is an allergic reaction to the strep infection and is most serious when the heart is involved. In these cases, the valves eventually become deformed and cannot close properly, a disfunction that impairs blood circulation through the heart. This valve destruction leads to, and is often diagnosed by, a permanent heart murmur.

LUPUS ERYTHEMATOSUS is considered by many doctors to be the gravest of the rheumatic diseases, although its symptoms vary greatly. It is a generalized disease of the connective tissues, and can affect (depending on its severity) joints, skin, the central nervous system, the blood, and internal organs.

The mildest form of lupus called *discoid lupus erythematosus*. This involves the skin only, usually on the face and neck, although the chest may also be affected. In its more severe form, the rash can be scaly and raised. The discoid form never involves internal organs. The rash is sensitive to sunlight, and can worsen after exposure.

The more severe from of lupus is known as *systemic lupus erythematosus* (SLE). SLE occurs nine times more frequently in women than in men, most commonly during the childbearing years. As with other types of arthritis, no one knows what triggers its onset, or why it will attack one member of a family and bypass others.

One of the difficulties in diagnosing SLE is that the initial symptoms are rather indistinct: fever, weakness, loss of appetite, weight loss, and synovial arthritis are common. It is this last symptom that confuses many doctors, as they mistake it for the cause of the other symptoms. This synovitis is different from typical rheumatoid arthritis, however, as the affected joints in a lupus patient may appear normal in X-rays. In fact, the synovial membrane is less inflamed than in true rheumatoid arthritis. Adding to the confusion between these two forms of arthritis is that they both affect virtually the same joints. Fortunately, the arthritis of lupus rarely causes any permanent damage. There is generally no damage to the joint, although on occasion there maybe some deforming, usually in the hands. Rather, the joint experiences a slipping (called a *subluxation*) due to a loosening of the tendons and ligaments. This condition causes discomfort but rarely disables the patient.

SLE is considered to be an autoimmune disease (see p. 2), with the arthritis of lupus being a manifestation of the body's reaction against its own tissues. Similarly, these antibodies can affect the blood in one of several different ways: *anemia* (low red blood cell count), a decrease in the white blood cell count (called *leukopenia*), or a lowered level of platelets (*thrombocytopenia*). This last can lead to bleeding, as platelets are essential in the clotting process. In severe cases of lupus, the antibodies may cause *nephritis* (inflammation of the kidneys).

Other parts of the body that may be affected in serious cases of SLE are the tissues surrounding the heart (pericardium) those surrounding the lungs (the pleura), and those surrounding the abdominal cavity (peritoneum), which may become inflamed.

ANKYLOSING SPONDYLITIS (also called Marie-Strumpel disease after the two doctors who first described it) is less well-known to the general public and has proven difficult to diagnose, in part because of doctors' lack of familiarity with it. The inflammation in this disease occurs at the locations of ligament and tendon attachments to the bones—the inflammation is *next to* the joint rather than *in* the joint, as in rheumatoid and osteoarthritis. The inflammation of AS causes stiffness and movement can become painful. This disease affects the central part of the body, particularly the spine. It is sometime referred to as "poker spine" disease, as it can cause fusion along the vertebrae, thereby making the patient hold his or her back stiffly, often at odd angles. Most often the initial area involved is the sacroiliac area of the spine, where the bottom of the spine is attached to the pelvis. After a while, often years, the stiffness and irritation begin to move up the back.

Although the spine is the prime target, pain in the back area and/or swelling in the joints are frequently the first signs of trouble. Many people ignore what they believe to be simply a stiff back for years, until more troublesome symptoms develop. Sufferers often go undiagnosed for as long as 20 years.

Complications in severe cases (which are very rare) of this disease include a recurring *acute iridocyclitis* (eye inflammation), widening of the aortic valves, and a condition called *amyloidosis*. This last is a condition in which the cells of the body undergo a gradual change that involves, in effect, a slow poisoning. The organs most often affected by amyloidosis are the liver, heart, and kidneys; their functions break down over time as the condition worsens. If the ankylosing spondylitis is discovered and treated successfully, however, these complications are unlikely.

Although there is no way to predict who will become an AS sufferer, research indicates that nearly all white AS victims possess a certain gene, called B27; while this gene also occurs in AS victims of other races, it is less prevalent in non-whites. Individuals who possess the gene B27 will not necessarily contract AS, but they appear to be at higher risk than those who do not possess the gene.

SCLERODERMA, like ankylosing spondylitis, is less well-known and, therefore, early signs are more likely to go undetected. The exact cause of scleroderma is unknown, but the condition stems from circulation disturbance in the small arteries. Areas of the body typically affected include the fingers, hands, arms, and neck. Initial symptoms include *Raynaud's syndrome*, which is a circulation cutback in the fingers and toes and is characterized by a change in skin color upon exposure of the affected areas to cold: the skin turns from its normal shade to first a blue, then a red shade. Not all people with Raynaud's develop scleroderma—indeed, most do not; it is simply, along with other symptoms, an indicator. Hardening of the skin is part of the process of the disease (scleroderma means, literally, "hard skin") for most patients. The degree of hardening differs from patient to patient.

Other parts of the body can be affected as well; difficulty in swallowing, for example, indicates involvement of the esophagus. The gastrointestinal tract, too, is often involved, with the most typical manifestations being dilation of the stomach and of the small intestine. The lower section of the lungs may be affected with scarring, and, rarely, kidneys may also suffer, with kidney failure the eventual outcome.

Scleroderma appears to be another of the autoimmune diseases, although this is still not a proven fact. The disease seems to manifest itself in middle age, with women affected more often than men. Scleroderma develops slowly, and it is not unusual for there to be long periods of remission.

LYME ARTHRITIS is another of the less well-known forms of rheumatic disease, although recent coverage of research in the press has brought it to the public's attention. It was first identified in the mid 1970s, after several cases occurred in the Lyme, Connecticut, area. The first symptom is a slowly spreading skin lesion, followed by headache, fever, and stiff neck. Later, the original symptoms may disappear, but they are almost always followed by joint abnormalities that closely resemble those of rheumatoid arthritis, cardiac involvement similar to that seen in rheumatic fever, and occasional neurologic irregularities.

One of the greatest problems in identifying the disease when it first came to doctors' attention was that the symptoms varied greatly among the patients. Furthermore, with remissions and flare-ups occurring unpredictably, doctors had no way of knowing whether or not the disease had run its course. Eventually, the "cause" of the disease was isolated: a tick bite triggered an infection which led to the onset of the arthritis. Further research into Lyme arthritis has yielded evidence that there has to be a genetic predisposition in the patient, as well as the "trigger" (the infectious agent), for the development of certain severe aspects of the disease. This may well be a helpful clue for further investigation into the mechanics of Lyme and other forms of arthritis.

PSORIATIC ARTHRITIS is one of the forms of rheumatic disease; it occurs in approximately 10% of all psoriasis patients, yet is little known by the general public. Psoriatic arthritis is a combination of inflammation of the synovium and of the ligaments and tendons. It is a relatively mild form of rheumatic disease, tending to affect the patient in very specific areas only, not causing the generalized weakness and stiffness of rheumatoid arthritis or SLE. Psoriatic arthritis usually manifests itself asymmetrically. Like osteoarthritis, it affects the end joints of fingers most often, but it is more capricious, affecting random fingers.

Of course, psoriasis is part of the disease, and the discomfort of that condition is part of the total picture. The scaly patches of thickened skin that are typical of psoriasis are present in psoriatic arthritis, and doctors find that treatment of the psoriasis itself can help the arthritis in some cases. It does, in this sense, seem to be linked specifically to the psoriasis.

Of all the rheumatic diseases, psoriatic arthritis seems to have the largest variety of possible symptoms, making it difficult to diagnose. Beyond the typical symptoms, there are some that are unusual; these are generally found in more serious cases. One, called *sausage digit*, occurs when there is swelling in both of the joints and the surrounding tissues in a finger or toe. In this syndrome, the affected finger or toe swells along its entire length, often to double its normal size, causing it to resemble a sausage. Another less common symptom is pain in the heel, which may come and go. In almost all cases of psoriatic arthritis, the skin problems are far more severe than those of the joints. One exception is a condition called *arthritis mutilans*, which is extremely rare (fewer than one in a thousand psoriatic arthritis patients develop this). It is said to be the most crippling and deforming form of arthritis, but it can be prevented if caught early and treated correctly.

REITER'S SYNDROME, first described by a German doctor (Hans Reiter), is relatively rare, although it is the second most common cause of arthritis in young men. Similar to ankylosing spondylitis in that the inflammation occurs at the juncture of ligaments and tendons to the bone, Reiter's syndrome differs from AS in that Reiter's affects the limbs and extremities more than it affects the spine. There is a similarity to psoriatic arthritis, too, in that in Reiter's the joints are affected randomly, rather than with the uniformity of rheumatoid arthritis.

Certain symptoms of Reiter's are present in all its victims: arthritis, eye inflammation, and a urinary tract discharge. The arthritis tends to be asymmetrical, and usually involves only a few joints at most. The swelling known as sausage digit (see psoriatic arthritis) can occur in Reiter's, too. Most likely to be affected are the feet, most typically the heel. Heel pain is usually located at the site of the Achilles tendon attachment or at the very bottom of the heel, where the arch ligaments attach to the heel bone.

The eye irritation associated with Reiter's is *conjunctivitis* (what many people call "pink eye"), which is an inflammation of the membrane that covers the inside of the eyelids and the tissue in front, under the eyeball. Most often only one eye is affected. There are cases in which the inflammation is deeper within the eye; this causes pain when looking at bright light and can even disturb the patient's vision. The urinary tract discharge (*urethritis*) is relatively innocuous, causing virtually no pain at all.

Another characteristic symptom, a skin rash called *keratoderma blennorrhagica,* occurs only in some cases of Reiter's syndrome. It is different from the rash of psoriasis, and appears most often on the palms and on the soles. The skin in these cases is scaly and red, but without the itch so common in psoriasis.

The progress of Reiter's syndrome is best described as episodic: it comes and goes, each attack distinct from the prior one. Some patients have only one or a few attacks in their entire lives, whereas others experience more frequent recurrences as time goes by.

Strong evidence suggests that Reiter's syndrome is caused by an infection, which may precede the onset of symptoms by several weeks. Two general types of infection may be responsible—one caused by a sexually-transmitted bacterium and the other by an intestinal bacterium which causes diarrhea. With the first type, contraction of the infection is followed by the urethritis; the other symptoms develop later. The other type develops after a bout of serious diarrhea, often long in duration. Research has shown a definite correlation between the bacterium responsible for Shigella dysentery and that responsible for Reiter's, but the presence of the bacterium alone does not mean Reiter's will necessarily develop.

As with ankylosing spondylitis, many Reiter's sufferers possess gene B27.

BURSITIS is a very common, self-limiting form of rheumatic disease, temporary in nature. A *bursa* is a small sac containing a lubricating fluid, found between a tendon and the bone over which the tendon glides, or between a ligament and the bone. Its function is to reduce friction as the tissues move over the bone(s). When the bursa becomes inflammed, either because of overuse of a joint or from a rheumatic disease, bursitis is the result. The pain is localized, and is greatest when the affected area is used. Redness and a hot sensation are also common. Most cases will ease on their own over the course of a few days to a week or so.

If, however, the action that brought on the bursitis is repeated, the condition will either never clear up entirely, or at least, recur. It is not a serious condition, though, and will not lead to crippling. Bursitis can be brought on by any number of activities that place stress on the same joint repeatedly. Tennis, baseball, and other joint-stressing sports are common causes, as are some forms of manual labor.

TENDINITIS is another common, self-limiting, localized rheumatic condition and is the result of overusing, or straining, a tendon, thereby causing it to inflame. It is most likely to result from exercise, although a rheumatic condition in the body can bring on tendinitis. As with bursitis, tenderness during use is the predominant symptom, and the affected part may feel warm, or even hot, to the touch.

CARPAL-TUNNEL SYNDROME is yet another localized, self-limiting condition. The median nerve, which travels into the hand to the muscles of the thumb and fingers (except the pinky), enters the hand through a structure called the *carpal tunnel*. This is an opening between the small bones at the base of the palm and a fibrous structure that bridges these bones. The median nerve is surrounded in the carpal tunnel by the tendons that flex the fingers.

When the nerve is pinched and/or squeezed, carpal-tunnel syndrome results. The symptoms are a pins-and-needles feeling in the thumb and all fingers except the pinky, shooting pain (either into the hand or up the forearm), numbness, and even a weakness of the thumb. The nerve is, in effect, inflamed from excessive pressure. This can happen as a result of rheumatoid arthritis, too much use of the wrist (from sports, for example), trauma to the wrist, or just leaning against a bent wrist too long. The condition does clear up with proper treatments, and only in the rarest of cases does it do permanent damage.

FIBROSITIS is another rheumatic disease that does not directly affect the joints. Rather, the target here is any of the deeper tissues in the body, most often in and around the muscles. The name means "inflammation of the fibers," referring to the fibrous coverings of the muscles. Doctors often specify MYOSITIS if the aching is specifically within the muscles. A person afflicted with fibrositis feels a general aching throughout the body. Symptoms are often more pronounced upon awakening, and may be made worse when the victim is chilled, tense, fatigued, depressed, or physically overworked in any part (or parts) of the body. Interestingly, fibrositis sufferers tend to share a history of inadequate exercise. One of the positive aspects of this condition is that it is not a progressive, destructive one. On the other hand, it can be difficult to diagnose and therefore does not always receive proper treatment immediately.

In recent years, doctors have identified three characteristic symptoms of fibrositis: general aching, a disturbed sleep pattern, and *extreme* tenderness in normally tender spots of the body. A partial profile of most fibrositis sufferers indicates an underlying tension problem. The victim is unable to relax the muscles (especially non-voluntarily), leading to increased soreness at spots that are tender even under normal conditions. This tension ties in with the sleep disturbances that are typical of fibrositis; the individual's muscles do not get the kind of rest (even during sleep) that they need. Electroencephalogram (EEG) readings of fibrositis victims differ from normal EEGs, demonstrating graphically the decreased slow-wave activity (physically the most restful kind of sleep).

The condition is not disabling and if treated correctly, it disappears, sometimes after only a few weeks.

POLYMYALGIA RHEUMATICA is the condition that most people refer to as "rheumatism." The name means "rheumatic pain in many muscles" and that is exactly what the condition is. Although the major complaint is the muscle ache, recent research suggests that the pain is caused by inflammation of small arteries that bring blood to the muscles. Arterial inflammation had been known to be a feature of more serious cases, but its identification as a potential root of the condition, regardless of the degree of severity, is more recent. The disease can become serious if left untreated; the stiffness and severe aching in neck, shoulders, and hips that typify the early stages can be joined by synovitis, exhaustion, low-grade fevers, and even noticeable weight loss. In extremely rare cases, the eyes will be affected (or, more precisely, the arteries leading to the eyes), and blindness can result.

The disease, left untreated, seems to last from three to five years, during which time the patient will have experienced most, if not all, of the symptoms, blindness included. On the other hand, treatment clears up the disease in a short time.

POLYMYOSITIS is an inflammation of the muscle and leads to actual muscle destruction. A profound weakness is the predominant symptom: not only does the victim have difficulty moving, but such basic functions as swallowing solids, talking clearly, and even lifting the head from a prone position become difficult. A related disease, DERMATOMYOSITIS, involves the skin as well as the muscles, and in childhood the muscle weakness is especially severe. Adult polymyositis victims who suffered childhood dermatomyositis are prey to a condition in which calcium deposits replace the destroyed muscle tissue, limiting motion even more severely.

When the skin is involved, blood vessels dilate and cause the skin in the affected area to change color noticeably (it takes on a purplish tinge). Internal organs may be affected, there may be a rash over large parts of the body, and Raynaud's syndrome (see

p. 8) may affect the fingers. Involvement of the lungs can lead to particularly serious problems, such as an inability to breathe vigorously enough or a tendency to swallow foods into the trachea. The disease, like so many of the rheumatic diseases, affects people differently, and to varying degrees.

Infectious arthritis refers to a number of forms of arthritis that are caused by infections and can be alleviated by treating the infection responsible. Three primary bacteria groups responsible for infectious arthritis are *staphylococcus, gonococcus,* and *tuberculosis bacteria.*

The arthritis of a staphylococcus infection is acute. It develops rapidly and is quite severe. Infected fluid in a joint causes it to swell, redden, and feel hot to the touch. The pain can be quite severe, and the victim will have a fever. In really severe cases (usually those left untreated initially), depending on exactly which staph germ is responsible, destruction of tissue within the joint can be quite rapid, and infection can spread to the other parts of the body, including the bone next to the original infected joint.

GONOCOCCAL ARTHRITIS is caused by the same bacteria that causes gonorrhea and seems to result after that disease is introduced in the body. This form of arthritis is much more prevalent in women than in men (some statistics show it to be 10 times more prevalent), probably because gonorrhea is easier to detect in the earlier stages—and thus is treated sooner—in men than it is in women. Gonococcal arthritis tends to invade the knee most often, but can affect several joints at once. The pattern of involvement is a scattered one, with joints on both sides of the body affected simultaneously.

Among the symptoms are genital discharge, characteristic blisters, fever, and abdominal pain. One strong indicator is inflammation at the back of the wrist. When that occurs with any of the more specific symptoms, gonococcal arthritis should be suspected.

TUBERCULAR ARTHRITIS is almost extinct now that tuberculosis is controlled. The most common form, once seen with great frequency, is tuberculosis of the spine (*Pott's disease*). Tubercular arthritis is a very slow-growing disease; the resultant symptoms differ greatly from those of the acute staph or gonococcal forms of arthritis. In tubercular arthritis, the joint is rarely hot and reddened. Another difference is that the swelling does not crop up so suddenly as in the other infectious arthritis forms.

Tubercular arthritis is more likely to affect the larger joints than the smaller. If the infection goes undetected for a long period, cartilage can be destroyed. When this happens in the hip or the knee, permanent disability can result.

2

DIAGNOSIS

Diagnosis of the specific form of arthritis you may be suffering from can be a long and involved process. To the traditional doctor, specific diagnosis is critical, and treatment can vary markedly according to the form of arthritis diagnosed. The alternative practitioner is less interested in the specifics, as he or she is likely to take a more holistic approach to your health. The same dietary or other form of treatment will probably be tried regardless of your specific symptoms or form of arthritis. This is based on the theory that if the condition of your body as a whole is improved it can then use its own resources to combat disease.

Many of the patients who seek help from alternative sources have already been through complete testing by traditional doctors and either are not satisfied with the results of treatment or are concerned with the potential side effects of invasive therapies. The test results and specific diagnosis may or may not form part of the basis for choosing a particular alternative treatment, but they are available if needed.

Diagnosing any of the rheumatic diseases involves several procedures. First, the doctor you have selected will examine your medical history and conduct a thorough physical examination. This part of the total procedure is very important; there are a wealth of clues to be found in what you have to say. For example, if the end-knuckles of your fingers are hurting (but not yet swollen), the chances are that you have osteoarthritis. The doctor will also want to determine when stiffness occurs and when it eases. With rheumatoid arthritis, for example, morning stiffness that eases after the victim rises and moves around is typical. Telling the doctor your particular symptoms very carefully is of major importance.

Your personal medical history may shed further light on the diagnosis by indicating family disease patterns. For example, several rheumatic conditions have been proven to have a genetic component. Others, although not yet proven to be genetic, are more likely to be contracted by individuals whose families have a history of occurence. It will matter to the doctor if a parent and a sibling have osteoarthritis, or if several female relatives on your mother's side have lupus. These facts may not be conclusive, but they certainly give your doctor diagnostic clues which are especially helpful with a disease that, for example, is as complicated to diagnose as lupus is.

Sometimes early physical manifestations such as restricted joint mobility can be detected by an experienced doctor; in such cases the general sense of what to look for (or what to suspect) may be narrowed somewhat. You may not be aware of certain habits you have developed in order to compensate for joint pain. A doctor is more likely to see the significance of stiffness, or a limb being held in an awkward way. With ankylosing spondylitis, for example, the sensitivity in the sacroiliac region, or a stiffly held back would certainly point to the final diagnosis. Similarly, skin conditions can be telling. Certain rashes are sometimes manifestations of rheumatic disease, especially lupus and psoriatic arthritis. You may not notice the lupus rash in its early stages, especially if you've been in the sun a lot (it could be mistaken for a suntan), but the doctor will certainly see it and recognize its significance. Added to other symptoms, the rash is like the final (or nearly final) piece of the puzzle.

Next in the diagnostic procedure is blood and urine testing. Not all tests are specific to a particular rheumatic condition, nor are the tests always positive at first. Taken with other physical findings, however, these tests can be quite useful in determining the severity of the disease, even in cases where symptoms are mild, and can serve to confirm a diagnosis. Many cases do not require blood tests, as physical findings and symptoms may be so clear that testing would be a waste of time and effort, not to mention money.

The variety of tests extends beyond just blood cell counts and urine analysis. There are blood tests for checking chemical functions of the body, others for identifying microbiological factors, and a blood test that shows the presence (or absence) of a genetic factor implicated in certain rheumatic diseases. Biopsies (analysis of tissue samples) may be performed to confirm diagnoses, or the fluid from a joint may be analyzed to determine what form of rheumatic disease is causing the inflammation. The full list is lengthy, and many of the tests are used only in rare cases. What is important is that you have some understanding of what your doctor is looking for, and why. Don't hesitate to question your doctor about the purpose and meaning of these tests. There is some disagreement about the validity of some of the more complicated tests, and there is even disagreement about test frequency. If you have your doubts, ask.

The tests described below are those used most frequently.

BLOOD TESTS

The blood counts useful in diagnosing rheumatic diseases are: the hematocrit, the white blood cell count, the differential white blood cell count, the platelet count, and the sedimentation rate.

The *Hematocrit test* is a measure of the total number of red cells in the blood. The RBC (red blood count) is affected by inflammation and will decrease in cases of chronic inflammation. This is useful in distinguishing between disease and a strained muscle or joint, for example. Another use for the hematocrit is to check the effects of drug therapy. Certain powerful medications have a negative effect on the bone marrow, where blood is produced; a reduced hematocrit is of tremendous significance in these cases.

The hematocrit is used to diagnose, or to confirm a diagnosis of, rheumatoid arthritis, lupus, and polymyalgia rheumatica.

The *White Blood Cell Count (WBC)* is just that; its significance is as an indicator of infection (white blood cells are the body's major defense against infection). An elevated WBC can be useful in determining if the particular form of arthritis is infection-related. Like the hematocrit, the WBC is important in monitoring the progress of certain drug therapies.

The WBC is useful in the diagnosis of lupus and infectious arthritis.

The *Differential White Blood Cell Count* checks the status of the five forms of white blood cells that are used by the body to combat infection. The test can be useful when there is infectious arthritis, but has its primary importance as a check on the progress of the more potent anti-malarial and immunosuppressive drugs used to treat some forms of arthritis.

The *Platelet Count* measures the level of platelets (also called thrombocytes) in the blood. The platelets are produced in the bone marrow and are used in blood clotting. A low platelet count can indicate a negative reaction to a drug, and is fairly typical of lupus.

The *Sedimentation Rate* (also called the erythrocyte sedimentation rate: erythrocytes are red blood cells) is used to measure inflammation. The test is very straightforward: blood is placed in a test tube and allowed to settle. The rate at which it settles is an indication of inflammatory activity, with higher rates pointing to higher degrees of inflammation. The test is not used specifically for any one disease, but will show the relative severity of any inflammatory disease.

The sedimentation rate is useful in tracking the progress of rheumatoid arthritis, juvenile rheumatoid arthritis, lupus, and polymyalgia rheumatica. In this last condition, the sedimentation rate is higher than in any other rheumatic disease.

The *Rheumatoid Factor* test (sometimes called the *latex* test) measures a substance in the blood called rheumatoid factor. A high count of rheumatoid factor may be indicative of rheumatoid arthritis. A high count alone, however, is not definitive evidence and must be supported by other test results and symptoms to be conclusive. The mere presence of the rheumatoid factor is no indication that the disease exists; it is the level that is important. This test may also be used in diagnosing lupus.

The *Antinuclear Antibody (ANA)* test, like the rheumatoid factor test, is not in itself conclusive. Antinuclear antibodies are produced in the body and are active against the nuclear material of the victim's own cells. Although people without lupus may have positive ANA tests, almost all lupus patients have these antibodies. A positive test can confirm lupus if other, less definite, symptoms are present.

The *Anti-DNA* test, like the ANA test, is used to diagnose lupus. DNA is a nuclear component of all body cells, and presence of the DNA antibodies almost always means the patient has lupus. The level of these antibodies in the blood indicates the severity of the disease.

BLOOD CHEMISTRY TESTS

Blood chemistry tests show the level of by-products from chemical functions in various parts of the body and, thus, how well the body is functioning. There are well over 20 such functions to be tested, but this discussion is limited to the four that are of use in diagnosing or monitoring various rheumatic diseases.

Creatinine levels in the blood indicate kidney function. It is not a test to diagnose a particular disease; rather, it serves to indicate the severity of kidney involvement in lupus.

Fibrinogen is a plasma protein, and levels will be elevated in polymyalgia rheumatica. This test, therefore, in conjunction with other findings, may be useful for diagnostic purposes.

Creatine phosphokinase is a muscle enzyme; when blood levels of this substance are higher than normal and other symptoms are present, either polymyositis or dermamyositis is the likely cause.

Aldolase, like creatine phosphokinase, is a muscle enzyme. It, too, when found at above-normal levels in the blood, points to polymyositis or dermamyositis.

BLOOD TEST FOR GENETIC FACTORS

Genetic factors may be determined by a blood test in which the white blood cells are typed. Such tests are of increasing interest and value to rheumatologists, among others. Presence of certain genes in the chromosomes indicates a predisposition for specific diseases. When certain symptoms point to a particular rheumatic condition, but are not conclusive, this test can confirm the diagnosis.

B27 is the name for a gene that is clearly associated with ankylosing spondylitis and Reiter's syndrome, and increasingly with psoriatic arthritis. If a person has the B27 marker he or she has close to a 20% chance of developing the disease. If the gene is not present, the odds are excellent that the person doesn't have AS. As this is a genetic component, children of AS patients can be screened and will know in advance whether to be on the alert for early symptoms of the disease. When caught and treated in the early stages, AS is not a serious problem.

The situation is practically the same for Reiter's syndrome. As both a diagnostic and screening tool, testing for the marker is invaluable.

Three marker genes, D4, D7, and D10, are linked to rheumatoid arthritis. This disease can be truly devastating in its severe stages; using the test for the appropriate markers can result in an earlier diagnosis and, in turn, earlier treatment to prevent serious disabilities.

URINE TESTS

The various compounds in the urine are important in some cases for diagnosis and in others for tracking the progress of drug therapy.

The presence of *red blood cells* in the urine can indicate inflammation of the kidneys, and in diagnostic testing such a finding would add weight to a verdict of lupus, which often affects the kidneys. When the disease has already been diagnosed and the patient is undergoing treatment with one of the potent antimalarial or immunosuppressive drugs, presence of blood in the urine is an indication that the drug may be too toxic; tests must be run to determine the course to take.

Proteins may also be found in the urine. As with finding red blood cells, the discovery of proteins may indicate kidney inflammation—and, therefore, lupus—at the diagnostic stage. When drug therapy has already been established, proteins in urine, like red blood cells, may well indicate serious side effects that may necessitate a change in therapy.

Uric-acid levels in the urine are very important when diagnosing and treating gout. Sometimes these levels are tested by means of a *24-hour urine sample*. As the name indicates, all urine excreted in a 24-hour period is collected, then the actual test for the required substance is performed. This method, although more inconvenient for the patient, is more accurate than the testing of a single urine sample. The 24-hour urine sample is also used to test for protein levels.

JOINT-FLUID TESTS

Joint-fluid examinations are very useful tests for diagnostic purposes. Fluid is withdrawn from the joint (the knee is the easiest to tap) and examined in one of two ways: microscopically and by culturing. Each has a distinct application.

Microscopic observation of joint fluid will show conclusively whether the disease is gout or pseudogout. Each of these is characterized by the presence of particular crystals in the synovial fluid. Uric-acid crystals, which are long and spiky, indicate the presence of gout. In pseudogout, the crystals are calcium pyrophosphate, which are basically square in shape. This procedure is also used when the doctor suspects, and wants quick confirmation of, infection as the cause of the attack. In the case of infection, the joint fluid will show greatly elevated levels of white blood cells which are used by the body to fight invading bacteria.

Once the presence of infection has been confirmed, the joint fluid will be cultured. In this process, the fluid is placed in a sterile growth medium; after a day or two the offending organism will have grown sufficiently to ensure a positive identification. The culturing is essential, for without an exact knowledge of which bacterium is present, the doctor cannot prescribe the proper antibiotic.

BIOPSIES

Biopsies are tests in which tissue samples are taken from a given part of the body and analyzed for specific characteristics. Skin, organs, muscles, arteries, and so on, all may be biopsied.

Skin biopsies are of use in diagnosing lupus, scleroderma, and psoriatic arthritis. The procedure, performed under a local anesthetic, is simple and safe. A small piece of the affected skin is lifted from the patient's body. The skin is then examined under the microscope for specific indicators that would confirm a diagnosis.

Muscle biopsies, although a bit more difficult to perform than skin biopsies, are equally safe. This test is essential for a conclusive diagnosis of polymyositis or dermatomyositis. If either of these is suspected, the doctor will select the weakest muscle to sample. This will ensure that the biopsy will show diseased tissue (not all muscles are affected, especially in the early stages of these two diseases). The muscle biopsy is also used to determine arteritis (inflammation of the arteries), as these blood vessels are present in muscles throughout the body.

Arterial biopsies are used in specific cases only. These are polymyalgia rheumatica (PMR) and a variation of PMR called giant-cell arteritis. The latter occurs when, as part of PMR, the patient suffers arterial inflammation, particularly in the head. Although the idea of an arterial biopsy seems very dangerous, the artery most often used for the procedure is the temporal artery, which runs in front of the ear and across the scalp. This is easy to reach and has the additional benefit of being just one artery in a rich network of blood vessels in the scalp. The procedure really is quite safe and can be very useful in arriving at a proper diagnosis.

X RAYS

X rays are less useful for diagnostic purposes than almost any other tests; they show only the bones, no soft tissues. Only rarely will bone damage be evident in the early stages of disease, and even when it is, there are usually other, more obvious symptoms to go by and diagnostic tools available that are equally, if not more informative. The only form of arthritis in whose diagnosis X rays play an essential role is ankylosing spondylitis; they have a coordinate function with other testing in the cases of psoriatic arthritis and pseudogout.

No diagnosis of ankylosing spondylitis is considered complete or conclusive without an X ray of the sacroiliac joints. These joints, at the bottom of the spine, show characteristic AS changes between 18 months and two years after the onset of the disease (most AS patients are not even aware of their disease at this early a stage). What happens is that the joints begin to merge, and an X ray shows a narrowed space between them. If the disease is more advanced than two years or so, the area shows a single bone; all joint space is gone.

In psoriatic arthritis, there is a tendency for new bone to grow on the sides of other bones. The new bone has a distinctive appearance on an X ray, because the new bone cells are not quite as dense and are not formed in a recognizable bone shape.

With pseudogout, there are usually calcium deposits on the cartilage of affected joints. Although the cartilage itself does not show up well, if at all (one exception is if it is inflamed, for affected tissue is denser than normal), the calcium deposits on the cartilage will be quite clear. This proof, in conjunction with the synovial fluid examination, serves to confirm the diagnosis.

X rays are, however, quite useful in checking the progress of disease. The one caution here is that too frequent use of X rays can be dangerous. Radiation has a cumulative effect on the body, with cell death, or chromosomal damage, among the more serious side effects. Therefore, your doctor should be careful and selective in ordering X rays. The procedure will be of most value when it can help give information that is not otherwise available. The most approrpriate use, by almost anyone's standards, is to indicate the type and extent of surgery required.

3

TRADITIONAL TREATMENT: MEDICATION AND SURGERY

Treating the various forms of arthritis is usually an involved, long-term process. The many elements of treatment must be considered as a whole, for it is only when all aspects are balanced for the individual that there is a real chance for relief.

PATIENT EDUCATION

Perhaps the first element to consider is patient education. So many doctors mention this as part of their treatment program that it must be considered a real form of therapy. It is often difficult for a patient to comprehend the long-term nature of rheumatic disease and the degree of its potential impact on the patient's future day-to-day life. This is both good and bad; if your particular case has an acute onset, or if the initial symptoms are severe and/or frightening, the idea of chronic illness can be overwhelming and can lead to depression. On the other hand, if you have less severe symptoms, and do not appreciate the implications of your disease, there is a chance that you will be too casual in following some of the more common-sense aspects of treatment.

You should, of course, be told what the disease is, how it affects the body, and what to expect in terms of immediate symptoms and immediate restrictions. For some patients, just being able to identify their malady is a major relief.

Such factors as rest must be discussed thoroughly. In most of the rheumatic diseases, rest is essential, but too much rest is detrimental. Your doctor should help you to design a proper exercise program.

If the particular condition warrants, medications will be prescribed. The role of drugs in rheumatic disease treatment is vital, and the patient must understand just what the drugs can and cannot do.

Understanding all of the general concepts of rheumatic diseases, as well as the particulars of your case, is an essential step in any treatment plan. Be aware that your doctor is there in part to answer questions. If a particular doctor rushes you, or doesn't give satisfactory answers, you should firmly request either more time or clearer, more definitive answers.

Some of the most important questions have to do with what to look for: dangerous symptoms, side effects from medications, how to differentiate between illness-related pain and pain that may be coincidental. Such information is vital to the patient, especially as treatment progresses. It is true that, as a patient becomes more familiar with his or her particular disease and its effects, he or she will know the answers to certain questions without having to call the doctor. That is good, but no one can reach that point without guidance and direction from a physician.

One item of importance in almost any form of rheumatic disease is weight. Too much weight adds stress on the hips, knees, ankles, and spine, and will certainly aggravate any existing arthritic condition in these areas. At the other end of the spectrum is undesired weight loss. This is almost always an indication that something somewhere is wrong, but it is very important to remember that when arthritis is present, weight loss is usually correctable. See your doctor immediately if weight loss occurs. Treatment for the underlying cause is always easier and more successful if caught early.

LIVING WITH DISABILITY

Coping with the disability that can result from arthritis is another area of tremendous importance. This is especially so in learning to do those everyday tasks which were once easy. These problems generally should be dealt with in consultation with a physical or occupational therapist rather than one's doctor, but there is no hard and fast rule about that. There *is* a need to compensate for the loss of certain abilities; fortunately, there is a considerable amount of information available on this subject. Various devices have been invented and manufactured to help affected individuals manage the tasks of dressing, opening drawers or jars, picking things up from the floor, etc. The most current information on these devices, as new ones are developed all the time, can be obtained from your local Arthritis Foundation chapter (see p. 127).

The specific treatments for the diseases will be discussed below. Do remember that every person is different and that each case of any given disease follows its own pattern. The treatments, as discussed here, are generalized programs that take into account the wide range of variations within each illness. The medications are described in some detail in the section following the one below.

TREATMENT APPROACHES TO DIFFERENT FORMS OF ARTHRITIS

Rheumatoid Arthritis This disease requires a treatment consisting of several factors: rest, exercise, occasionally physical aids, and medication. The basic goal is to reduce inflammation and, therefore, the potential for joint destruction. Resting a joint will help, but too much rest stiffens joints. Your doctor, or a physical therapist, will be able to suggest specific exercises and appropriate frequency of repetition. A patient may find the use of braces, splints, or even a cane or crutches beneficial at any given time to ease a joint that is especially painful. In such cases, exercise is especially important; if the joint in question is immobilized it will stiffen.

Medication will be an integral part of any treatment program for rheumatoid arthritis. Aspirin (p. 27) can be the only drug ever needed; nonsteroidal anti-inflammatory drugs (p. 27) are the next most powerful drugs; gold salts (p. 33) and penicillamine (p. 33) are even stronger than the anti-malarials. Corticosteroids (p. 31) can be beneficial, although the medical profession seems unable to agree whether, in fact, these potent drugs are appropriate for rheumatoid arthritis. Similar controversy surrounds the use of immunosuppressive drugs (p. 38), which can have extremely hazardous side effects. (It is important the user to remember that all these drugs serve the purpose of reducing the symptoms of inflammation and pain and are not curative.)

Surgical treatment may include total hip or knee replacement (p. 44), synovectomy of the knee or knuckles (p. 42), and metatarsal head resection (p. 43).

Plasmapheresis and cryofiltration (p. 40), although experimental, are used in some cases and may be valuable.

Osteoarthritis Exercise is important in treating osteoarthritis. The disease is only slowly progressive, and exercise will help maintain joint function. Most doctors recommend walking, but some prefer swimming because the body is supported by water, which thus reduces stress on the weight-bearing joints. As with rheumatoid arthritis, there may be times when a cane or some other form of physical aid will help alleviate pain, but the temptation to become reliant on the aid must be avoided.

Medications used are aspirin (p. 27), nonsteroidal anti-inflammatories (p. 27), and occasional corticosteroid injections (p. 32).

Surgical treatment may include total hip or knee replacement (p. 44).

Gout Treatment for gout may involve dietary changes to eliminate those foods and beverages high in uric acid, and a carefully planned and monitored program of medication.

In an acute stage, the goal is to reduce the inflammation. Colchicine (p. 37) is the most commonly prescribed drug for this, but sometimes one of the other anti-inflammatories (p. 27) is preferred.

In the period between acute episodes, there are several drugs that reduce the uric acid levels in the body (p. 36). In addition, there are various urinary alkalinizing agents (p. 38) which make the uric acid more soluble, thus speeding its excretion from the body.

If the patient has *chronic tophaceous* gout, either probenecid (p. 36) or allopurinol (p. 37) is used.

Pseudogout Treatment for pseudogout includes exercise (swimming is a good, gentle, all-over exercise) along with medication. The most effective drugs are the nonsteroidal anti-inflammatories (p. 27). Colchicine (p. 37) may be of some value. Sometimes steroid injections (p. 32) into the joint are beneficial. Surgery is unusual; there are rare cases when a hip or knee will be replaced.

Juvenile Rheumatoid Arthritis Exercise (swimming) and physical therapy are especially important for patients with this condition, since most will outgrown the disease and muscles must be maintained.

Medications are used with great caution in treating this disease. Aspirin (p. 27) is the primary component of drug therapy, but must be monitored. Most of the nonsteroidal anti-inflammatories are specifically designated as being unsafe for children. Corticosteroids (p. 31) are rarely used, and then only for short-term treatment, as they can prevent bone growth. Surgery, although atypical, would most likely be synovectomy of the knee (p. 42).

Systemic Lupus Erythematosus If severe, this disease requires more careful monitoring of activities than most other rheumatic conditions. The sun can aggravate skin symptoms and, accordingly, may need to be avoided in varying degrees. Rest, too, can be important. Anxiety can cause flare-ups of symptoms, so situations that provoke it should be avoided.

Medications depend on the extent of the illness. Drug therapy may include only aspirin (p. 27). Any one of the various other drugs, from the nonsteroidal anti-inflammatories (p. 27) through the immunosuppressives (p. 38), may be called for at a given time during the progression of the disease. In addition, if internal organs are affected, medicines may be prescribed to correct or ease those problems.

Only rarely is surgery indicated for the arthritic conditions in SLE. Those instances are usually limited to total hip replacement (p. 44) after severe damage has already taken place.

Plasmapheresis and cryofiltration (p. 40) are still considered experimental, but hold great promise for lupus patients.

Ankylosing Spondylitis Exercise is especially important to AS patients. It is essential to counter the tendency for bone fusion, especially along the spine and neck, that is the hallmark of this disease. This is accomplished by stretching on a daily basis. Additionally, special deep-breathing exercises should be included to stretch apart the ribs and retard fusion there. Posture exercises, too, are an important part of the regimen.

Although aspirin (p. 27) may be used, the nonsteroidal anti-inflammatories (p. 27) usually provide substantially better results.

Scleroderma In the case of this disease, exercise is required primarily for the purpose of stretching the skin, but it also serves to improve circulation. Basic common-sense is called for in some situations: if the patient suffers from Raynaud's syndrome, for example, keep the hands and upper body warm.

Lyme arthritis   The general precautions and guidelines recommended for rheumatoid arthritis apply here, as the arthritic involvement most closely resembles typical rheumatoid arthritis.

The drug therapy for this infectious form of arthritis depends on severity. Aspirin (p. 27) can be beneficial; if not, the nonsteroidal anti-inflammatories (p. 27) should bring relief. (Remember, these are usually not to be used for children.) Corticosteroid injections (p. 32) in the knee (one of the most frequently affected joints) are administered when severe inflammation does not respond to more conservative drugs.

Psoriatic arthritis   Patients with this condition need to exercise the joints to avoid progressive stiffness, as in rheumatoid arthritis.

Although there are similarities between psoriatic and rheumatoid arthritis, the medications most often prescribed differ. The nonsteroidal anti-inflammatories (p. 27) tend to be more beneficial than aspirin (p. 27). The corticosteroid (p. 32) and gold salt injections (p. 33) are controversial in that both can ultimately increase the psoriasis that is part of this disease. Immunosuppressives (p. 38) have been used to advantage in severe cases.

Reiter's Syndrome   Similar to ankylosing spondylitis in several respects, this disease is treated with careful exercise of the affected areas to maintain mobility, and with a program of medication.

Most often nonsteroidal anti-inflammatories (p. 27) are prescribed. This disease can be difficult to treat with these particular drugs, yet your doctor is more likely to stay with them than go on to more potent therapies, none of which seems as useful. If there is eye involvement, corticosteroids (p. 31) are usually administered.

Bursitis   This local condition is treated most often by patience; time is the best healer of all, here. Some exercise is valuable to prevent stiffening, but it should not be continued to the point at which it causes real pain. Heat, too, will help ease the discomfort. If the condition has not cleared itself after several weeks, a doctor should be consulted. If the condition is severe, nonsteroidal anti-inflammatories (p. 27) or even a corticosteroid injection (p. 32) into the inflamed area might be indicaated.

Tendinitis   Like bursitis, this condition can best be cared for by a balance of rest, intelligent limited exercise of the affected part, and time. Medications are not very effective and the use of painkillers can prevent you from knowing when you've over-used the injured area. If there is no improvement after several weeks, your doctor should be consulted. There may be need at this point for a nonsteroidal anti-inflammatory (p. 27); corticosteroids (p. 31) are used only in very rare cases, when the other forms of treatment are not effective. (Too many of these injections near the inflamed tendon can actually harm the tendon.)

Carpal-Tunnel Syndrome   Treatment for this condition almost always involves stabilizing the wrist. There is a special wrist splint that will keep the hand in the best position for healing. Your doctor may prescribe a nonsteroidal anti-inflammatory (p. 27), but that is for quite severe cases only.

Fibrositis   Daily exercise is the single most important part of treatment. It is beneficial both physically and emotionally, as it relieves the tension that is so much a part of this disease. Any other activity that will help the patient relax and sleep better is desirable. Drugs, on the other hand, do not help.

Polymyalgia Rheumatica The treatment for this condition is limited to medication. Most often corticosteroids (p. 31) are prescribed and offer immediate relief. There is a rather long maintenance period on this drug, but the results are worth it. Some doctors prescribe aspirin (p. 27) or a nonsteroidal anti-inflammatory (p. 27) for mild cases.

Polymyositis and Dermatomyositis The treatment is the same for both, and is likely to vary depending on your doctor. Some physicians feel that exercise actually adds to the symptoms, whereas others believe that the exercise encourages muscle strength and maintenance. There is no single truth here, so part of the decision should rest with what feels right to the patient. Gentle exercise may actually make the patient's emotional state more positive, which can only help.

Medication is nearly always restricted to the corticosteroids (p. 31), and continues for quite some time. There are patients whose disease does not respond well to the steroids; immunosuppressives (p. 38) may be of help in these cases.

INFECTIOUS ARTHRITIS

There is no typical treatment for infectious arthritis, as treatment is determined by the particular infectious agent causing the disease.

Staphylococcal and Gonococcal Arthritis These are treated with antibiotics. In both kinds of arthritis, the patient is usually hospitalized initially in order to institute and monitor the proper administration of the drugs (intravenous injections). Drainage of the affected joint is indicated in cases of severe infection and inflammation; it is more common in staph infections than in gonococcal infections.

Tubercular Arthritis This condition is treated by antibiotics specific to the bacterium that causes the infection; drainage of joint fluid depends on individual need. If such need exists, the drainage procedure may be repeated over a period of time. Medication is administered orally (which obviates the need for hospitalization) and continues for up to a few years. This seemingly long term of treatment is related to the nature of tubercle bacilli; they may remain alive but inert for some time, only to become suddenly active under conditions of stress. Too limited a treatment increases the chance of recurrence.

SPECIFIC MEDICATIONS: ADVANTAGES AND SIDE EFFECTS

Medications will, in most cases, be used for long periods, which makes the sensible course to follow that which uses the least potent drugs possible. The stronger drugs tend to have stronger, and more dangerous, side effects. Also, a patient can develop resistance to the positive effects of a medication, necessitating strong drugs as time goes by. So, even though it *is* necessary to reduce inflammation and ease pain, it is equally necessary to be prudent. A side note on the easing of pain: if too strong a drug is taken, the patient will not feel the pain at all, and may end up damaging the affected joint(s) further through overuse.

Aspirin   A salicylate, aspirin is the most basic anti-inflammatory drug in the arthritis arsenal. Its ability to serve as both an anti-inflammatory agent and an analgesic qualifies it as the drug of choice for most forms of arthritis. As an anti-inflammatory, it reduces the swelling of the affected tissues; this is the major goal in treating synovitis and many other rheumatic conditions. Its ability to ease minor pain is an added value. What is critical in prescribing aspirin is the dosage. The analgesic and anti-inflammatory properties differ greatly: 10 grains (two adult aspirin tablets) every four hours is the perfect analgesic dosage, but bare minimum for the anti-inflammatory needs. In rheumatoid arthritis, for example, most doctors would prescribe twice that amount to relieve the inflammation adequately.

Aspirin can cause side effects. The condition of a person taking high dosages should be monitored so that any side effects can be evaluated against the benefits and the dosage adjusted accordingly. Among the side effects of aspirin are ringing in the ears, stomach pains and/or nausea (which may indicate the formation of stomach ulcers), lightheadedness, and/or headaches (!). Appearance of any of these when taking aspirin is a signal to review the dosage with your doctor. A general rule of thumb with aspirin in treating rheumatoid arthritis is that the most effective dosage for a patient is that which is just below the point at which side effects begin.

There are other forms of aspirin available. Some are buffered with antacids, which ease the stomach irritation commonly associated with plain aspirin. As prolonged treatment with aspirin can cause stomach ulcers, it is a good idea to check with your doctor to find out whether a buffered aspirin would be better. Some aspirins are coated with a substance that reduces the irritation of the stomach lining. Unfortunately, the coating can also cause the aspirin to be absorbed less completely through the stomach, thereby giving less relief. Other aspirins are available in a time-released form, which spreads out the dosage over a set period of time. This may ease some of the stomach problems, but will not necessarily do so. Most of the fancier forms of aspirin are considerably more expensive than plain aspirin and may not be any more effective.

Remember that aspirin *is* a drug, despite its availability and familiarity. Be aware at all times of exactly how much aspirin you are taking (if your doctor has left that up to you) so that you will be able to discuss dosage in the event of side effects or complications. Treat aspirin as respectfully as you would a prescription medication.

NONSTEROID ANTI-INFLAMMATORY DRUGS

There is another class of drugs, called Nonsteroidal Anti-inflammatory drugs, which may be used in those cases where aspirin has proven unsuitable. One of these may be ideal for individuals who truly cannot tolerate aspirin and its side effects. For the most part, these drugs are less likely than aspirin is to cause stomach problems. They are not, however, without hazards or drawbacks. There is no common chemical ground among all these medications (as is the case with the salicylates), and it is quite possible that certain patients may be sensitive to some component of them, with resultant bad reactions. There may be a need to try different drugs among this group to find out which works best for a particular patient.

Ibuprofen **(trade name: Motrin)** Ibuprofen can produce gastrointestinal side effects similar to those associated with aspirin (irritation of the stomach lining, nausea, heartburn), but because it is absorbed well after eating, some of these problems may be forestalled. It may cause peptic ulcers and/or gastrointestinal bleeding in some individuals. Fluid retention, too, can be a problem, as well as rash, and/or dizziness.

Give ibuprofen at least a week to begin working; if your condition has shown no noticeable improvement by then, let your doctor know. It may be wise to switch medications in that case. Ibuprofen may be used in combination with gold salts and/or corticosteroids, but not with aspirin. Its use and effectiveness for children has not been established.

Naproxen **(trade name: Naprosyn)** This has one advantage over many of the other nonsteroidal anti-inflammatories, which is that its effects last longer and, therefore, fewer pills per day are required. The side effects are less severe, and less frequent than with aspirin, but they do exist. Gastrointestinal bleeding can be severe; peptic ulcers, too, have been reported. Other complaints are nausea, headaches, dizziness, ringing in the ears, itching, and fluid retention. Another side effects may be a blurring or reduction of vision, and impairment of color perception has sometimes been noted; if any one of these symptoms occurs, it is very important for you to have a thorough ophthalmologic examination.

Naproxen may be given in combination with gold salts and/or corticosteroids, but does not seem to enhance the effect of the corticosteroids to any great degree. This drug should not be used with aspirin or given to children, for whom its safety and efficacy have not yet been established.

Naproxen sodium **(trade name: Anaprox)** This is very similar to Naproxen, to which it is related. The most frequent side effects are heartburn, nausea, headaches, dizziness, ringing in the ears, and fluid retention. It is not clear whether Naproxen sodium is less likely to cause peptic ulcers than aspirin is. The warning above concerning Naproxen-related eye trouble also holds for Naproxen sodium. To be safe, an individual undergoing prolonged therapy with this drug should check with an ophthalmologist periodically.

Fenoprofen **(trade name: Nalfon)** This drug is capable of producing the gastrointestinal side effects common to aspirin, ibuprofen, and naproxen, but seems to do so less frequently. Fenoprofen has not been shown to cause any adverse eye reactions. However, it is wise to have a thorough check-up periodically to be sure, since this drug is part of the family of nonsteroidal anti-inflammatories, some of which do affect the eyes. Fenoprofen can cause genitourinary tract complications, primarily cystitis and blood in the urine.

Safety and effectiveness for children have not been determined, so it should not be prescribed for them. As with ibuprofen, after one week's treatment some real benefit should be discernible. If not, check with your doctor.

Tolmetin Sodium **(trade name: Tolectin)** This drug can cause the same side effects as the other nonsteroidal anti-inflammatories, although less frequently. Nausea is the single most frequent reaction, with headaches next on the list. There is no reported incidence of eye involvement, but because of the adverse eye reactions associated with other nonsteroidal anti-inflammatories, it is wise to have your eyes checked periodically.

Tolmetin can be given with steroids and is also of use in juvenile rheumatoid arthritis. In that disease, the benefits and side effects are very similar to those of aspirin.

Phenylbutazone (**trade name: Butazolidin**)   This is one of the two earliest drugs developed for specific anti-inflammatory purposes. (The other, oxyphenbutazone, is discussed below.) Over the last twenty years or so, certain dangerous side effects have been attributed unquestionably to continued use of phenylbutazone, specifically *aplastic anemia* and *agranulocytosis*. These are both serious blood conditions: in aplastic anemia, the bone marrow is poisoned and the formation of both red and white blood cells is suppressed. Agranulocytosis is the total absence of granulocytes, which are the white blood cells that spring into action against acute infections. Granted, few patients are afflicted with these side effects, but the risk is one that must be considered. The usual gastrointestinal side effects can be present in patients using phenylbutazone, as well as fluid retention. As with ibuprofen and fenoprofen, a one-week trial will serve to indicate whether the drug will work for a given patient. If a long-term program is planned, expect frequent blood tests to check for signs of the blood conditions described above.

Oxyphenbutazone (**trade name: Tandearil**)   This drug is so similar to phenylbutazone that the only further information given here concerns preference. Of the two, oxyphenbutazone seems to be prescribed more often because it is slightly (but only slightly) less likely to cause stomach upset.

Indomethacin (**trade name: Indocin**)   This drug can cause depression, dizziness, headaches, and/or a slightly unfocused, disoriented sensation, as well as the usual stomach problems. The head symptoms may disappear as the body becomes accustomed to the medication. If they continue after the first two to three weeks, check with your doctor, who may want to switch medications. This is another of the drugs whose benefits should be apparent by the end of the first week. If there is relief of inflammation but the head symptoms persist, you and your doctor will have to evaluate the total situation and decide whether you should remain on indomethacin.

A time-released formulation of this drug has just recently been suspended from the market in several foreign countries out of concern over reports of negative side effects from the drug. The U. S. Food and Drug Administration is still considering the identical form for approval here. The suspension does not affect the regular form of indomethacin.

Indomethacin should not be administered with aspirin, and needs to be monitored when given concomitantly with probenecid (p. 36). This need arises from the tendency of serum levels of indomethacin to rise in the presence of probenecid (used in treating gout). Also, indomethacin has not been proven either safe or effective for children under 14, and should not be prescribed for them.

Sulindac (**trade name: Clinoril**)   Fewer pills of this drug are required per day than is the case with most of the other nonsteroidal anti-inflammatories. Otherwise, it is quite similar to the others. Peptic ulcers and gastrointestinal bleeding have been reported occasionally, and gastrointestinal pain is not uncommon. The drug also can cause dizziness, headache, and rashes.

Sulindac may be given in conjunction with corticosteroids and with probenecid (for gout), but not with aspirin. There are no firm data on safety or effectiveness for children, although studies on sulindac's use for juvenile rheumatoid arthritis are under way.

ANTI-MALARIAL DRUGS

The *anti-malarial drugs* are another group of medications used in treating rheumatic diseases. Although they were developed to control malaria, they serve also to control inflammation. The medications, synthetic derivatives of quinine, are cumulative in effect, building up slowly in the body. This means that several weeks can pass before the positive effects of the drugs are noticeable; similarly, the compounds disappear from the body slowly and may continue to exert their influence after the patient stops taking them.

The primary side effect of these drugs is eye damage, both corneal and retinal. If caught early, the corneal changes are reversible once the medication is stopped. Retinal changes are not so easily reversed, and in some cases blindness results; this happens extremely rarely, however, and only after long-term treatment. Doctors prescribing these drugs should insist on ophthalmologic exams at the beginning of treatment (to provide a base-line for future comparison) and every three months thereafter.

There are other possible side effects, including muscle weakness, psychosis, and blood disorders. Less serious side effects include such gastrointestinal symptoms as nausea, diarrhea, and abdominal cramps; central nervous system involvements such as irritability; weight loss; and lassitude. Most of the side effects, including those affecting the eye, seem to be dose related.

The anti-malarials are not seriously risky, despite these warnings. They are compatible with both corticosteroids and salicylates; when taken together with anti-malarials, the corticosteroids and/or salicylates can be decreased gradually, or even eliminated, once the anti-malarials have been used for a few weeks and begin to help.

There is one anti-malarial, it must be noted, that is *never* to be used for arthritis patients, according to its manufacturer. That is Aralen Phosphate (a brand of chloroquine phosphate) with Primaquine Phosphate. The reason is that many arthritis patients have a tendency to granulocytosis, a shortage of granulocytes (a type of white blood cell), which can be caused by this medication.

It is wise, if pursuing a long-term treatment with any of the anti-malarials, to have periodic blood counts taken. These will alert your doctor to any blood changes that are unusual for your disease and, thus, may be drug-related. Any findings that cannot be attributed to the disease itself would indicate a need to change drug therapy.

The anti-malarial drugs used to treat arthritis-related conditions are:

Chloroquine Hydrochloride (Aralen Hydrochloride injection)
Chloroquine Phosphate (Aralen Phosphate)
Hydroxychloroquine Sulfate (Plaquenil Sulfate)

Plaquenil Sulfate is the only one of these drugs that is indicated by the manufacturer for acute or chronic rheumatoid arthritis (although the others are used, this seems to have the best all-around "track record"). The manufacturer also states, as do the others, that if "objective improvement" (easing of stiffness, for example) is *not* noticeable within six months of treatment, use of the drug should be discontinued.

CORTICOSTEROIDS

The next most powerful drugs, going up the spectrum, are the *corticosteroids*. These synthetic formulations produce effects that are the same as, or similar to, those of natural hormones. Like hormones, these drugs have the ability to suppress inflammation and allergic reactions, and they also affect various chemical processes in the body. These qualities are like double-edged swords, however: inflammation is a necessary part of the body's defense system, reacting against infection and injury; if it is suppressed completely, the body is left without a valuable defense mechanism. Yet, as described in Chapter 1, too much inflammation can cause real destruction, especially in the enclosed area of a joint; thus, some means of control is necessary. Similarly, although corticosteroids are needed to affect certain chemical processes in a positive way, continued administration of "therapeutic" doses can result in serious problems.

Another side effect, potentially more serious, is that continued doses of corticosteroids serve to curb the activity of the adrenal cortex. It is as if the cortex gets the message that there are enough of these compounds in the body, and it need not continue to work. Unfortunately, cessation of this natural activity leaves the patient without any cortex hormones if medication is stopped abruptly. Thus, if it becomes necessary to discontinue corticosteroid treatment, the patient must be weaned from the drugs over a period of time in order to allow the cortex to resume its proper functioning; even then, there is the risk that full function will not return.

The safest use of oral corticosteroids is on a short-term basis. Only rarely do any side effects occur if the treatment lasts for a week or less. After about one month of corticosteroid treatment (especially if the dosage is a high one), any of the following may occur: ulcers, infection, and fluid retention with the accompanying "moon face" and elevated blood pressure. As the treatment continues beyond that time, other, more radical effects may develop: diabetes is possible; bone and fibrous tissue become weak, leading to possible fractures from normally minor falls or injuries; psychotic behavior can be manifested; healing processes are less efficient;

and the torso thickens from increased fluid retention. The adrenal glands can cease functioning, as described above, although it is nearly impossible to state definitively at what point this will happen.

Another way to minimize the effects of corticosteroids is to inject them directly into the affected area. Such local application usually is saved for acute flare-ups that do not respond well to other medications. The actual procedure must be done with extreme care, so that the needle is placed precisely into the synovial fluid, not the surrounding tissues. The reason for this is that there can be cellular damage if the steroid is injected into tissue. An additional point to be aware of is that most pharmaceutical companies warn that corticosteroids should not be injected into unstable joints.

Another form of treatment involves the administration of *adrenocorticotropic hormone* (ACTH). A natural hormone formed in the pituitary gland, ACTH stimulates the adrenal cortex to produce natural corticosteroids. If the adrenal cortex is healthy, this treatment can be useful. The major danger here is that, if treatment is repeated too frequently (and, as with the adrenal cortex, the critical moment is impossible to predict accurately), the pituitary gland will cease production of ACTH, leaving the body without this essential hormone.

The consensus about ACTH is that it should be used only if other treatments have proven ineffectual, and then only in acute episodes. Even so, the U. S. manufacturer of ACTH states that these medications have "limited therapeutic value in those conditions responsive to corticosteroid therapy." One of the biggest difficulties with ACTH treatment is that, although the amount of ACTH in the dosage is known, there is no correlation between that dosage and the amount of natural corticosteroids produced in response. Most doctors prefer to know exactly what dosage of corticosteroids is in action against the patient's disease. There are many detrimental side effects from treatment over a long period of time, and there can even be some immediate, allergic-type reactions to ACTH treatment. Doctors considering using ACTH should test patients for porcine protein sensitivity if it is suspected, as the formulation of ACTH used involves these compounds.

All in all, the management of the use of corticosteroids is tricky, at best. There is no agreement on what situations call for the use of these drugs or on what constitutes a proper dosage, so that each doctor must rely on experience and individual judgment. Most physicians will prescribe the drugs only after a more conservative treatment has been tried and found unsuccessful. Do not hesitate to discuss this treatment with your physician if it is recommended. The side effects can be extremely serious, and even though there may be no other medication your doctor feels will work for you, you should explore all aspects of steroid therapy and feel that the decision is the right one.

Several oral corticosteroids are identified below (generic names will precede brand names).

Cortisone (**sold only by generic name**) This drug is rarely used now because, in addition to sharing the side effects associated with other corticosteroids, cortisone retains fluid, thus adding to the potential problems.

Hydrocortisone (sold only by generic name)   This drug poses the same problems as cortisone.

Prednisone (Deltasone, Meticorten, Orasone, SK Prednisone, Sterapred Uni-Pak, and generic name)   The prednisone family drugs are liable to cause any or all of the side effects of corticosteroids. Follow your doctor's orders *to the letter,* as dosage strength and frequency can affect the onset of side effects. Many doctors feel that prednisone is the oral steroid of choice, because it is less expensive than the others as a result of being available in generic form, and serves the same purpose as the other oral corticosteroids.

Triamcinolone (Aristocort, Kenacort, SK Triamcinolone, and generic name)   The triamcinolone drugs are fluorinated steroids. Muscle-wasting, one of the side effects of long-term steroid use, tends to be more severe with fluorinated steroids (when they are taken orally) than with other types, making them less desirable than, for example, the prednisone group. The manufacturers of Aristocort claim it causes less sodium (salt) retention than other corticosteroids.

Dexamethasone (Decadron, Dexone, Hexadrol, SK Dexamethasone, and generic name)   These, like the triamcinolones, are fluorinated steroids, and have the same tendency to cause muscle-wasting. As a result, they are generally less desirable than prednisone. The manufacturers of Hexadrol claim that this product causes less salt and water retention than other steroids.

Methylprednisolone (Medrol)   Methylprednisolone is chemically more similar to prednisone than to the others, and therefore more closely resembles it in both effect and side effects.

GOLD SALTS AND PENICILLAMINE

Two other drugs, similar to one another in effect, are used in the treatment of rheumatoid arthritis, lupus, and psoriatic arthritis— gold salts and penicillamine. Both are far more potent, in their benefits and in their side effects, than the corticosteroids. Many doctors consider these to be innovative drugs, perhaps because both remain controversial. They are used only when other, more conservative treatments have already been tried unsuccessfully. Both can produce truly serious side effects.

Gold salts have been used in treating rheumatoid arthritis since the 1920's, despite their potential danger, because they can be extremely effective. If administered at an early enough stage, before cartilage and bone have been damaged, they can bring about an actual remission of the disease. If treatment is begun at a later stage, when destruction has already set in, the gold salts can prevent further damage but cannot reverse the course of the disease.

Gold salts and penicillamine both work on a cumulative basis, meaning that the benefits of treatment take some time to become noticeable: two months is average. Similarly, the effect of the drug lingers on after treatment. Not surprisingly, therefore, the most serious side effects tend to develop once treatment is well-established. However, certain allergic reactions to the gold salts can occur at *any* time during treatment. These include fainting, swelling of the tongue, difficulty in breathing and/or swallowing, and anaphylactic shock. This last is rare, and occurs when the allergic antibodies throughout the system are connected to the tissue (normally they are in the bloodstream). Presence of the allergen (gold salts in this case) activates these antibodies systemically; air passages are compressed, and blood pressure drops precipitously. There is insufficient blood flow through the brain, and the condition can be fatal. Probability of allergic reaction can be determined by test injections one or two very small doses given before full treatment begins. These tests can point out allergies by bringing on slight reactions, thus making it possible to avoid exposing the patient to the full-blown allergic symptoms a full dosage could have produced.

More probable than these allergic reactions are other side effects. They range from dermatitis (skin inflammation, almost always itchy) to severe blood disorders and kidney damage. The list is long, and includes involvement of nearly every system of the body. Because of the definite possiblity of blood and/or kidney reactions, it is essential for blood and urine analyses to be run prior to the initiation of treatment. These will provide base-line readings against which your physician can compare future tests, which should include a urine analysis before each injection and complete blood and platelet counts every two weeks. Either or both of these procedures will allow any damage that may occur to be spotted at its earliest stage and halted by discontinuing treatment with the drug in question. If caught early, the side effects mentioned are nearly always reversible.

Other, less obvious side effects can signal trouble before it has been spotted in the urine or blood test results. Even something as seemingly benign as itching, slight nausea, dizziness, a sore mouth, or a metallic taste in the mouth should be reported to your doctor at once, as these are among the side effects that might indicate an intolerance to the medication; treatment should be monitored carefully while tests are taken to determine whether these reactions are from the medication.

One possible transient effect of these injections is arthralgia (literally "joint pain"). If it occurs, it may last a day or two following the injection. It will ease, and the presence of such an effect is not usually reason enough to stop treatment. Your doctor may want to stop temporarily to see whether the arthralgia disappears quickly; if it does, treatment can be resumed.

Gold salts are one part of a total treatment program. They may be used with aspirin or other salicylates, and even with the non-steroidal anti-inflammatories, except for phenylbutazone and oxyphenbutazone. Like gold salts, these two can cause severe blood disorders, as noted earlier. Gold salts should *never* be used in combination with penicillamine, anti-malarials, or immunosuppressive drugs. It must be noted here that a sizable number of patients (nearly 25% according to estimates) who try gold salt therapy have to stop because of side effects. In such cases, penicillamine may be the next drug tried.

Penicillamine, a synthetic derivative of penicillin, is similar to gold salts in several ways: its action is cumulative; it, too, can actually suppress disease activity; and its propensity for causing serious and kidney blood disorders poses a serious threat to the patient.

Doctor and patient should weigh all potential benefits and risks carefully before beginning treatment with this drug. As with gold salts, base-line urine and blood analyses are essential, with follow-up analyses of urine prior to every injection and of blood and platelet counts every two weeks. It is also advisable when taking penicillamine to have liver function tests run every six months during the first year and a half of treatment, as there have been reports (albeit rare) of liver problems caused by the drug.

Penicillamine can also have other, less serious side effects: fever, sore throat, chills, bruising, and/or bleeding. The occurrence of any one of these should be reported immediately; your doctor can then determine whether the penicillamine is at fault and, if it is, can stop treatment. Like gold salts, penicillamine can trigger gastrointestinal reactions. In addition, it can cause the sense of taste to diminish. One of the rarer adverse reactions to this drug is a set of symptoms that appears to be an early stage of myasthenia gravis. Whereas myasthenia gravis is a progressive disease of the voluntary muscles, which become weakened, the reactive syndrome disappears when the medication stops.

Any patient who has a sensitivity to penicillin should avoid penicillamine since there is, theoretically, a strong probability of cross-sensitivity and, therefore, a great risk of severe allergic reaction. Even a patient with no sensitivity to penicillin may experience allergic reactions to penicillamine. In this case, the allergies are less serious than those associated with gold salts, but two distinct rashes may result. The more common of the two is a generalized, itchy rash that appears within the first few months of treatment. It usually disappears within days of medication being stopped and rarely recurs if treatment is resumed later. If necessary, this early rash may be eased by the administration of antihistamines.

The other rash—called a late rash—appears after treatment has been established for six months or more. It usually occurs on the trunk of the body and, unlike the early rash, is intensely itchy. Topical corticosteroids (cream or spray form) usually do not relieve it; generally, the only effective course of action is to discontinue the penicillamine. This late rash may linger for weeks, even after the medication is withdrawn, and will almost always recur if treatment is resumed.

A side effect that is unique to penicillamine (and, fortunately, is rare) is a lupus-like syndrome. Lupus erythematosus (see p 6), a rheumatic disease of the connective tissues, is also an auto-immune disease. It can be quite serious, but this medication-caused syndrome is not *true* lupus. Blood tests may mimic those of a lupus patient, showing a positive anti-nuclear antibody reading. This does not necessarily indicate that treatment should be stopped. Rather, your doctor should monitor this syndrome carefully, and review the decision about penicillamine periodically.

Another side effect peculiar to penicillamine is an increase in the amount of soluble collagen in the body. Collagen, a protein, is the major component of connective tissue. The effects of this condition may include longer healing time, weaker scar tissue, or unusual bruising at sites of physical stress (elbows, knees, etc.), where the skin seems to become less substantive. This condition generally is reversible.

Both penicillamine and gold salts may cause arthralgia. If this condition occurs, expecially in many joints simultaneously (polyarthralgia), your doctor may prefer to discontinue treatment long enough to determine whether the condition is a reaction to the medication.

Penicillamine can be administered concurrently with the salicylates, the nonsteroidal anti-inflammatories (except phenylbutazone and oxyphenbutazone, for the same reason gold salts should not be used with them), and systemic corticosteroids. *Never* use it in combination with gold salts, antimalarials, immunosuppressive drugs, or the two nonsteroidal anti-inflammatories mentioned above.

Gold salts are available in two formulations: gold sodium thiomalate (trade name: Myochrisine) and sterile aurothioglucose suspension (trade name: Solganol Suspension).

Pencillamine (trade names: Cuprimine, Depen Titratabs)

DRUGS FOR THE CONTROL OF GOUT

There is a group of drugs used specifically for treating gout, most of them because of their ability to control uric-acid levels. Some of the drugs act to speed uric acid excretion in the urine (these are called *uricosuric* agents), and others prevent the production of uric-acid. Another drug, *colchicine*, is neither a uricosuric agent nor a uric-acid preventor. Rather, it seems that colchicine reduces the inflammatory response to the uric-acid crystals that are deposited in the joints. It also minimizes the action of the white blood cells, which "flood" the affected joint in response to infection and add to the pain. Colchicine is rather specific in its applications, it is used either to stop an acute attack of gout or to prevent acute attacks during the interval period.

Probenecid (trade names: Benemid, SK Probenecid, and two generic brands) The most important thing to remember about this uricosuric agent is that treatment with it must begin *after* an acute attack has subsided. Aspirin is not to be given at the same time as probenecid, as it interferes with the action of the drug. If necessary, an acetaminophen (Tylenol and Datril are two brand names) may be substituted. Urine alkalinizing agents (p. 38) can increase the action of probenecid, and fluid intake should be increased while taking the drug. These two measures can prevent some of the potential side effects that involve the kidneys, such as blood in the urine and formation of uric-acid stones in the kidneys.

Other side effects of probenecid can include headaches, nausea, vomiting, itching, and dizziness, although the incidence of such reactions seems infrequent.

An often prescribed form of probenecid is one that is combined with colchicine (trade names: ColBenemid, and two generic brands). Probenemid by itself can bring on attacks of gout as the level of uric-acid lowers, and the addition of colchicine to the medication acts to prevent the acute attacks. As with plain probenemid, no aspirin should be administered; acetaminophen is a suitable replacement. Treatment with this combined medication, as with plain probenemid, should begin only after an acute attack has eased.

Sulfinpyrazone (trade name: Anturane)   This drug is prescribed to treat chronic and intermittent gouty arthritis only. It is not intended to relieve acute attacks. It is a powerful uricosuric, and patients using it are recommended to take alkalinizing agents (p. 38) and increase their fluid intake to help prevent kidney involvement. Aspirin and other salicylates block the action of sulfinpyrazone; an acetaminophen (e.g., Tylenol, Datril) may be substituted.

Side effects most often include stomach disturbances, so the manufacturers recommend that this medicine be taken with food, milk, or antacids. Severe nausea or vomiting usually indicates an overdose.

Colchicine (sold by generic name only, in both tablet and injection form).   This drug has an almost immediate effect when used to stop an acute attack. It can be administered either orally, or by intravenous injection. The problem with colchicine when used orally in acute attacks is that it usually causes abdominal cramps, nausea, vomiting, and/or diarrhea. If the reaction becomes severe (especially vomiting or diarrhea, which can lead to dehydration), stop taking the medicine and call your doctor. The intravenous injection carries little chance of the side effects, but a doctor must administer the injections.

When colchicine is taken for preventive purposes, the daily dosage is much lower than when the drug is used to combat acute attacks (pills are then taken hourly, as a rule), so side effects are virtually non-existent. When taken over a very prolonged period of time, however, colchicine may cause bone marrow depression. Your doctor may want to monitor its effect by running periodic blood tests.

Allopurinol (trade names: Lopurin, Zyloprim)   This drug reduces the production of uric acid by inhibiting the bio-chemical reactions that immediately precede the acid's formation. In this way, both blood serum levels of uric acid and the level of uric acid in the urine are reduced. In some cases kidney stones made up of uric-acid crystals can accumulate. When this happens, other problems than gout must be dealt with. Some doctors find it prudent to determine whether the uric-acid level in the excreted urine is normal or elevated. If it is elevated in a 24-hour urine sample (p. 18), allopurinol is prescribed to alleviate the condition (probenecid would be appropriate if the level were normal). Treatment should be continued for at least a week or more; if it is stopped too soon, the uric-acid level will return to its original elevated state.

Unlike probenecid, allopurinol may be given concurrently with aspirin, as salicylates do not affect it. *Never* combine allopurinol with either mercaptopurine (p. 39) or azathioprine (p. 39). The manufacturers do not warn specifically against such a combination, although they note that the two immunosuppresive drugs (p. 38) have a heightened effect in combination with allopurinol and, thus, should be taken in smaller doses when combined with it. However, there have been instances of fatality when either of the two was combined with allopurinol, and it is not worth taking the risk.

Typical side effects of allopurinol include skin rash, drowsiness, nausea, and vomiting. Other gastrointestinal effects have also been reported. It is important to stop taking allopurinol if a rash appears, because this condition can be followed by more severe reactions. Check with your doctor if you experience any of the reactions mentioned.

Various *urinary alkalinizing agents* may be recommended for patients taking probenecid (either by itself or in combination with colchicine) or sulfinpyrazone. Two of these are described below; a third, *sodium bicarbonate*, is also used, but it is more likely to cause the over-alkaline conditon noted as being a potential problem with the other two. The function of these solutions is to make the uric acid more soluable, thus speeding its excretion from the body.

Sodium citrate and citric acid solution (trade name: Bictira). This solution must be diluted and taken after meals. There may be an adverse reaction called alkalosis (an excess of alkali in the body), although it is rare with this solution. The urine can be tested for alkalosis; if necessary, the patient can stop taking the alkalizer.

Potassium citrate, sodium citrate, and citric acid solution (trade names: Polycitra syrup, Polycitra-LC) As with the sodium citrate solution, either of the two formats of the potassium citrate combination must be diluted and taken after meals. As with any alkalizing agent, there is some possibility of alkalosis; the urine should be monitored for this.

CYTOXIC AGENTS

The most powerful, dangerous group of drugs, called *cytoxic agents*, is sometimes used in extremely severe cases of rheumatoid arthritis, lupus, or on occasion, other forms of rheumatic disease. These drugs were originally intended to suppress or stop tissue growth, and represent part of the chemotherapy arsenal used in cancer cases. Another function they serve, it was found, is to suppress white blood cell growth, thereby affecting the body's immune responses; these drugs are also called *immunosuppressives*. One last application is to relieve conditions that seem to be, or are, autoimmune in nature. Lupus is such a disease, and although rheumatoid arthritis has not yet been proven to be an autoimmune disease, there is growing evidence that it is. The strength and potential dangers of these drugs are great. Any doctor considering one of these drugs for a particular patient must inform him or her of these dangers, and together they must agree that the benefits are worth the risks. The attitude held by many doctors is that these drugs still are experimental and thus must be reserved for only the most severe or seemingly hopeless cases of rheumatoid arthritis or lupus. Other doctors respect the power of the immunosuppressives, regarding them as part of the full spectrum of treatment available to all patients when conditions warrant.

Cyclophosphamide (trade name: Cytoxan) This is probably the most potent of the immunosuppressive drugs. The most typical side effect is leukopenia (shortage of white blood cells)—a side effect shared by all these drugs. Such cells are an important part of the body's defense mechanism, and a consequence of leukopenia is therefore an increased vulnerability to infection. If infections occur, it is wise either to modify the dosage or to interrupt treatment. Blood counts will usually return to normal if treatment is suspended. Blood counts, especially for the white blood cells, must be taken frequently throughout the full term of treatment.

A more dangerous side effect which is all too probable with this drug is a form of cystitis (inflammation of the bladder) caused by the concentration of poisonous residues of the medication. To prevent this, the manufacturer warns (as your doctor will remind you) that you should have "AMPLE FLUID INTAKE" (capitals theirs) and should empty your bladder frequently. If this cystitis does develop, treatment must stop. Blood in the urine should clear up within a few days after the medicine is withdrawn, but in rare cases it has been known to persist for several months.

More side effects are the gastrointestinal reactions of nausea, vomiting, loss of appetite. These, although common, seem to be a function of the dosage as much as of an individual's sensitivity. There may be hair loss (regrowth is expected when treatment ceases); skin and fingernails may darken; and the lungs may be affected by fibroid growths. This last is usually restricted to patients taking high doses for very long periods of time.

Less common, but highly serious, side effects are the suppression of normal activity of the ovaries or testes. This seems, too, to be dosage related, but may be irreversible in long-term treatment.

Azathioprine (trade name: Imuran)   This drug has sometimes proven effective in retarding the progress of rheumatoid arthritis. It is relatively well-tolerated, but can have serious consequences. Because azathioprine is capable of producing an irreversible depression of bone marrow function, the manufacturer suggests that complete blood and platelet counts be run "at least weekly," with more frequent counts taken during initial therapy.

The major side effect is lowered blood cell production. The action of this drug may be delayed; therefore, if the drop in the blood count is ususually large, it is wise either to reduce the dosage or to cease the medication, even if only temporarily.

Sometimes a patient may experience nausea, vomiting, diarrhea, or even anorexia. Mouth lesions, rashes, hair loss, or drug fever have been observed, and one of the side effects noted after a long-term treatment is liver damage. There is no bladder involvement as with cyclophosphamide, nor does azathioprine seem to affect the sex glands.

Mercaptopurine (trade name: Purinethol)   This is a drug whose immunosuppressive quality is similar to azathioprine's. It poses the additional hazard of potentially causing chromosomal damage, and women who take it during the first trimester of pregnancy have a higher than ordinary incidence of natural abortion. The drug also have a negative effect on fertility.

Mercaptopurine is more likely than azathioprine to cause liver damage. Gastrointestinal side effects are unusual during initial stages of treatment, but do seem to be symptomatic of toxicity from the drug. As with other immunosuppressives, frequent blood counts are required throughout the treatment.

Chlorambucil (trade name: Leukeran)   This cytotoxic drug carries fairly forbidding warnings from the manufacturer: severe depression of bone marrow function; presumption of carcinogenic potential; probably a mutagenic agent (affecting human chromosomes); and negative effect on human fertility. Yet, with this drug, the effect on bone marrow is considered "only moderate" at therapeutic doses, and this effect reverses quickly upon termination of treatment. Weekly blood counts are necessary to prevent irreversible damage, with more frequent white blood cell counts during the first three to six weeks. It seems that chlorambucil is more likely to produce blood changes in an unpredictable pattern, thus necessitating more frequent white blood cell counts.

Mechlorethamine (trade name: Mustargen) This was the first cytotoxic drug used experimentally for treating rheumatoid arthritis. It is similar in many ways to cyclophosphamide, and causes many of the same side effects. It is not often used today, but is still available. The possiblity of bladder involvement is great with mechlorethamine, and fluid intake should be maintained at high levels to combat this side effect. The drug is injected, and the manufacturer suggests administering the drug at night, in case sedation is necessary to help tolerate the side effects.

These side effects include nausea and vomiting, depressed levels of some of the white blood cells (especially the lymphocytes), development of infections (typical with immunosuppressive drugs), suppression of sex gland functions, and chromosomal damage.

If your doctor recommends mechlorethamine, check to find out why, and whether one of the other immunosuppressives might be better.

PLASMAPHERESIS AND GOLD ION INJECTION

There is another realm of treatment, considered by many orthodox doctors to be experimental at best, alternative (which carries a pejorative sense) at worst. This treatment is under investigation at several hospitals throughout the country, and is prescribed by many doctors for particular patients as a regular part of therapy. It is *plasmapheresis*, and there is a growing body of literature pointing to the benefits of this process.

Plasmapheresis is a non-surgical technique. Quite simply put, it is to arthritis what dialysis is to kidney disease. The analogy is not entirely accurate, but it does present a quick understanding of what is involved. The procedure (apharesis and plasma exchange are alternate names) involves the insertion of a needle attached to tubing in the patient's vein, from which the blood is taken. It flows through the tubing into a filtration machine, in which the plasma is separated from the red and white blood cells by centrifugal action. The patient's own plasma is discarded, and new fluids (either fresh-frozen plasma, or plasma products) are substituted and returned with the blood cells to the patient.

The purpose of plasma exchange is to remove those substances in the plasma that instigate, irritate, or somehow influence the course of the disease. In the case of rheumatoid arthritis, there are immune complexes and various proteins that seem to have some bearing on the disease; their removal can ease symptoms.

One of the major disadvantages of plasma exchange involves the quantities of plasma products required for replacement purposes. In a paper published by five doctors conducting research at Cleveland Metropolitan General Hospital's arthritis clinic (Drs.

James W. Smith, Kohji Kayashima, Yoshihiro Asanuma, and Yukihiko Nosé, and Paul S. Malchesky, M.S.), the authors state that if the procedure were found to have real benefit for patients with the disease currently under investigation, there would not be enough plasma available to treat everyone. (At that time, in 1982, more than four million liters of plasma were being collected annually in the United States.) The paper also identified complications that can arise from plasma or plasma products infusion.

The doctors reported on one procedure, a variation on the plasmapheresis technique, that has been developed in response to these complications. Called *cryofiltration* (cold membrane filtration), this procedure does not rely on centrifugal separation of plasma from blood cells; rather it employs two membrane filters. The first membrane filter separates the plasma from the blood; after this separation, the plasma is cooled (the tubing circuitry runs through an ice-water bath), then passes through a cooled membrane which separates the large molecules of immunoglobulins, various proteins, and other compounds, from the fluid. Next, the filtered plasma is returned to the blood flow (still in the filtration system outside the patient's body), warmed to body temperature, and returned to the patient.

Neither procedure is commonly available, and certain questions remain to be answered: Which patients will benefit most? Can successful results be predicted and if so, by what criteria? Which medications should be given concomitantly? How will all this be funded? There are still many unknowns. The research at the Cleveland clinic certainly points to the more positive effects of the cryofiltration system. The case for an even more sophisticated system, one that could filter out specific macromolecules responsible for a particular disease, is raised in the paper mentioned above. What stands in the way of such a system is that there is no clear knowledge yet of which substances cause irritation and disease. The advantages of the membrane filtration system make it worthy of further study. There is less blood cell loss, and the need for replacement plasma or plasma products virtually disappears, thus removing the risks that accompany plasma infusion.

There are hospitals where plasmapheresis is offered, and for those patients whose disease does not respond to the various medications, or for whom certain medications are not feasible, the procedure might be of value. You should not discount a procedure just because it is experimental. If it interests you and your condition warrants it, discuss plasmapheresis with your doctor.

A new method of treating rheumatoid arthritis and the equipment needed for that procedure have just been granted a patent by the federal government. Wilson Greatbatch, an engineer in Clarence, New York, has devised a means of injecting *gold ions* directly into an affected joint. The apparatus he designed consists of a gold electrode, a battery, and a current generator. The entire unit can be implanted within the patient's body, with the electrode attached to the diseased joint.

Once the circuit is complete and the current generator is working, the electrode gives off ions into the joint. Experimentation will be necessary to determine whether the new procedure can yield better results than other treatment approaches and, if so, with what side effects.

SURGERY

Various surgical procedures are used to help patients whose joints have been permanently damaged by arthritis. These operations can reduce or eliminate pain and significantly improve function. They are generally expensive, although eventually improved techniques and newer materials should lower the cost. Certainly the results can be worthwhile.

A few pieces of advice to follow when considering surgery seem almost to obvious to mention, but they are important and thus bear repeating. The first is to get a second opinion. Practically no surgical procedures connected with arthritis are life-threatening. Although many procedures are almost 100 percent successful, any surgery carries some risk. The second precaution is to have a truly competent orthopedic surgeon handling your case. The procedures are detailed, often quite delicate, and it is necessary to have someone performing your operation who is both familiar and comfortable with the specific surgical technique. Ask to whom your doctor would go for the same operation. Call other rheumatologists or internists to ask for their recommendation. And, most important, speak with the surgeon before you decide to have the operation. Get information about the procedure. Make sure that all your questions are answered. Do not let the surgeon (or, indeed, any other doctor!) bully or ignore you.

Ask both your doctor and the surgeon whether the planned operation has a high likelihood of success, i.e., of improving your condition and relieving pain. Sometimes surgeons will differ with non-surgeons in opinion. A rheumatologist or internist is likely to see the patient for a more extended period after recovery from surgery, especially if the patient obtains little or no relief from that surgery. If two doctors differ substantially in their opinions, get as much information as possible from both, or consult another surgeon or rheumatologist. Try to reconcile the varying opinions to your satisfaction before you decide to go ahead.

The operations themselves are quite varied. Some involve removal of tissues, others insert bone substitutes.

SYNOVECTOMY

Synovectomy is, literally, the removal of the synovial membrane. This procedure is usually performed when the inflammation of the synovium has proven uncontrollable by medication. There is still controversy among doctors regarding synovectomy. Some doctors claim it is, at best, a means of delaying symptoms of arthritis while others state that it effectively counters the progress of the disease.

Yet another part of the controversy concerns the question of when the surgery should be performed. There is some evidence that it offers greater relief if it is performed before any bone erosion has occurred, prompting some doctors to feel that surgery should take place during the earlier stages of the illness. Other doctors claim that it is wiser to wait because, if the disease is mild and relatively easy to control with medications, the rush to surgery will cause unnecessary discomfort and expense. They feel that the benefits of waiting outweigh the risk of bone damage prior to surgery. Still other doctors believe that any surgery, unless absolutely necessary in a life-threatening situation, is traumatic and should be avoided.

The synovium does grow back, with regeneration taking from six months to almost a year (although seven to eight months is generally considered to be average). The benefit from surgery comes during the period before the synovium grows back. In this time, the inflamed tissue and the enzymes it produces are not eroding the bone. The regenerated synovium can become inflamed, but most doctors have found that when this happens, the inflammation is less severe than before surgery.

This surgery is most often used for rheumatoid arthritis (involving the knee and finger knuckles). It may be used in severe cases of juvenile rheumatoid arthritis (where the knee is most likely to be the joint involved), Lyme arthritis (again, the knee), or psoriatic arthritis.

ARTHRODESIS

Arthrodesis (fusion) is the procedure in which a joint is fixed in one position. If the cartilage is stripped from the moving surfaces of a joint, the bone ends are exposed and can be joined together. The final effect is, surprisingly, a more mobile limb (or other part of the body). Prior to surgery, the patient may be afraid to use the arm, leg, etc., in question because moving it causes severe pain. Once the affected joint is fixed in position, the pain is eliminated. Another benefit is that the joint, before fusion, may be out of alignment and, as a result, pressing on nerves. The nerve involvement is relieved by fusion, thus ending another source of pain.

This procedure can be applied to fingers, wrists, ankles, and even vertebrae. A potential for future difficulties from this operation lies in the fact that an immobilized joint places stress on neighboring joints. They, in turn, may suffer damage over the course of time. Another problem with this surgery is that it may not be successful, (particularly when it involves joints that bear weight or absorb a great deal of stress).

RESECTIONING

Resectioning of a bone occurs when the bone is actually cut and part is removed. This procedure is one element of joint replacement (see below), but as an operation on its own, it has a particular application. Most often it is used in severe cases of rheumatoid arthritis, when the feet are involved and medication is not helping. The metatarsal bones are the five long bones that connect the ankle and heel to the toes (you can feel these bones at the top of your foot). The head ends of these bones (where the toes are connected) are removed, leaving the joints more mobile and less painful. Sometimes parts of the toe bones are removed as well, when the condition is severe enough.

JOINT REPLACEMENT

This general category of surgery is the fastest growing and most intensively researched of all surgical procedures used to treat joints severely damaged by arthritis. The ends of the bones are replaced by substitute joints (increasingly sophisticated versions are being developed continually, it seems), usually made of stainless steel or one of the more recently developed alloys. The replacement is usually glued in place with a plastic cement and a plastic substance in substituted for the cartilage.

This operation is receiving such attention because it, more than any of the other techniques used today, offers patients renewed mobility and freedom from pain. For those whose condition is severe and who have been handicapped by their disease, the opportunities to resume even a partly functional life are marvelous.

The joints replaced most frequently are hips, knees, and finger knuckles. There are experimental procedures and replacements being developed and refined for other joints, as well. The procedure is similar in all cases. The ends of the bones that enter the affected joint are removed. The implant for each bone end is cemented into place or in the case of finger knuckle implants, each end is inserted into the hollow finger bones on either side of the joint. If the implanted joint is made of metal, most often its surfaces will have a coating of plastic or silicone rubber. Finger implants are usually made entirely of a rubber or plastic. Any tendon problems at the joint are corrected at the same time the implant is inserted. As the area around the joint heals, fibrous tissue grows around the substitute, which helps to hold it in place.

There is a new advance in joint replacement which is still in the experimental stage. It is worth detailing here because it points to a new era of longer-lasting implants. A team consisting of two orthopedic surgeons, Drs. Kenneth Krackow and David Hugerford, and a designer, Robert Kenna, at Good Samaritan Hospital in Baltimore, has developed a porous knee. The surfaces of the joint are made of a porous alloy composed of chrome and cobalt. The porous quality of these surfaces allows blood to infiltrate, after which it clots. New bone grows onto the surfaces of the joint, bonding with the blood. Eventually this new bone growth will mature, and the knee will be established in place. There is evidence, after two and a half years since the first human application of this joint, that growth is following the anticipated pattern.

No joint replacement is guaranteed to last indefinitely, however. Most replacement knees, for example, last for four to seven years, with a second operation necessary when the first replacement finally loosens to the point of uselessness. Hips seem to last longer, no doubt because the joint is less complicated than a knee. A 10 year period of use from an artificial hip is average. Although the procedure, as with any surgery, will cause some discomfort and pain, the results provide remarkable improvement.

Operations to replace joints are used for patients with severe damage from rheumatoid arthritis, osteoarthritis, pseudogout (on occasion), lupus, and psoriatic arthritis. Lyme arthritis, too, can cause damage similar to rheumatoid arthritis; it is a disease for which this procedure should be beneficial in appropriate cases.

RECOVERING FROM SURGERY

Any post-surgical recovery requires teamwork between the patient and a variety of specialists, and length of recovery will vary from patient to patient. In addition to the surgeon and the referring rheumatologist or internist, physical and occupational therapists, psychologists or psychiatrists, and social workers all might have a particular role to play. It is of utmost importance that the patient know exactly what he or she may and may not do with the new joint.

Exercise of the joint, and of other parts of the body that may have been inactive prior to surgery, is essential, but such exercise must be tailored to the particular situation. The physical therapist can prepare an individualized program of movement and exercise for the patient. Once mobility and strength increase, the patient has to relearn to use the affected part of the body in a purposeful way, a process in which the occupational therapist can offer expert guidance. In many cases, too, the patient must readjust to being a mobile, functioning person after having been to a large degree incapacitated for a long period of time; counseling can do wonders to help a patient revive or develop a positive self-image. Lastly, but certainly of equal importance, is the role of the social worker, who can help the patient make the transition to the "outside world" in terms of finding a job, if work is once again possible, or finding out about services available to ease that transition.

ORTHODOX MEDICINE AND OSTEOPATHY

	Medications	Surgery	Exercise	Diet	Note
Rheumatoid Arthritis	Aspirin, nonsteroidal anti-inflammatory drugs, anti-malarial drugs, gold salts, penicillamine, and sometimes corticosteroids and immunosuppressive drugs	May include total hip or knee replacement, synovectomy of the knee or knuckles, and metatarsal head resection	Specific exercises and/or physical therapy		Rest to reduce inflammation, but not so much as to cause increased stiffness
Osteoarthritis	Aspirin, nonsteroidal anti-inflammatory drugs, and occasional corticosteroid injections	Total hip or knee replacement	Swimming or walking		
Gout	Colchicine and other anti-inflammatories; urinary alkalizing agents			Elimination of foods and beverages high in uric acid	
Pseudogout	Nonsteroidal anti-inflammatories	Unusual, but sometimes hip or knee replacement	Swimming		
Juvenile Rheumatoid Arthritis	Aspirin generally the only medication, as others have harmful side effects for children	Extremely unusual	Exercise program including swimming and physical therapy		
Systemic Lupus Erythematosus	Aspirin, nonsteroidal anti-inflammatories, immunosuppressives	Extremely unusual			
Ankylosing Spondylitis	Aspirin and nonsteroidal anti-inflammatory drugs		Stretching, deep breathing, and physical therapy		Avoidance of sun; rest; avoidance of anxiety

Scleroderma	Corticosteroids for muscle inflammation	Exercise to stretch skin and improve circulation	
Lyme Arthritis			Same general guidelines as for Rheumatoid Arthritis
Psoriatic Arthritis	Nonsteroidal anti-inflammatories tend to be more beneficial than aspirin. Immunosuppressives in severe cases	Exercise of joints to avoid progressive stiffness	Other than medication, similar guidelines as for Rheumatoid Arthritis
Reiter's Syndrome	Nonsteroidal anti-inflammatories. If eye involvement, corticosteroids	Careful exercise of affected area	Similar to ankylosing spondylitis
Bursitis	In severe conditions nonsteroidal anti-inflammatories, or corticosteroid injections	Exercise to prevent stiffness should be stopped if it causes pain.	Will often clear up by itself with rest; heat often helpful
Tendinitis	Nonsteroidal anti-inflammatories in severe cases	Exercise to prevent stiffness should be stopped if it causes pain.	Will often clear up by itself with rest
Carpal-tunnel Syndrome	Nonsteroidal anti-inflammatories in severe cases		Stabilization of the wrist
Fibrositis		Daily exercise very important	

ORTHODOX MEDICINE AND OSTEOPATHY (*Continued*)

	Medications	Surgery	Exercise	Diet	Note
Polymyalgia Rheumatica	Aspirin and nonsteroidal anti-inflammatories for mild cases, corticosteroids very helpful in more severe cases				
Polymyositis and Dermatomyositis	Corticosteroids. Immunosuppressive drugs may help in some cases.		Some physicians feel exercise is helpful; others feel it's harmful.		
Infectious Arthritis	Specific antibiotics determined by the cause of the infection	Drainage of the joint sometimes necessary			Patient may be hospitalized to ensure proper administration of drugs.

4

ALTERNATIVE TREATMENT

CLINICAL ECOLOGY

This relatively new medical discipline has expanded rapidly, both in its applications and in people's awareness of it, since it first began to take form in the late 1950s. The name Clinical Ecology emphasizes the importance of observing the mutual relationships between organisms and their environment; it can be said that this approach studies and treats life in its environment as influenced by its environment.

Clinical ecologists see patients whose illnesses are a direct result of something controllable in their environment, something that may well be other than bacteria or viruses. The science of clinical ecology really began when some orthodox physicians, prime among them Dr. Theron G. Randolph, began to perceive that allergies were not quite what they had studied in medical school.

These doctors gradually came to the conclusion that allergies can produce symptoms far more diverse than the itchy eyes, runny nose, and hives with which most people associate the term. Conditions as varied as headaches, exhaustion, urinary-tract infections, fluid retention, arthritis symptoms, depression, and even psychosis have been identified as allergic reactions. Moreover, these symptoms (among others) disappeared when the allergen (also called *excitant*—the substance to which the patient is allergic) was eliminated from the patient's environment. In addition, clinical testing could provoke the symptoms and the patient was as ill as if the original conditions had never been treated.

Clinical ecologists claim that many symptoms of mental and physical illness are symptoms of allergies. Because of this belief, they prefer to determine whether a patient's condition is a reaction to something in the environment before they recommend treatment by an invasive therapy. Simply to remove an irritant from the patient's environment at the very least does no harm; at the very best, it can solve real health problems. As clinical ecologists see it, to prescribe a drug is invasive; something is literally being forced into the patients "ecology," as it were. It is well known that all drugs can cause adverse reactions. Clinical ecologists, who are well trained as orthodox physicians, do not reject that form of medicine on all counts. Rather, they believe it is wiser and safer to withhold invasive therapy until other options have first been tried.

The question arises at this point: If, in fact, the beliefs of clinical ecologists are reasonable and true, how do they determine to what substance(s) a patient is allergic? The possibilities, of course, are virtually unlimited. An interesting aspect of clinical ecology is that a person can conduct testing for allergies alone, without a doctor. The methods by which a clinical ecologist would conduct such tests differ slightly from those which someone without similar training would use, but the theory is identical.

Clinical ecologists have found that real hints are found in a person's eating and drinking habits. Very often the foods or beverages you crave the most are the ones that are most responsible for your symptoms. It is thought by more and more clinical ecologists that these foods and drinks may, in fact, be addictive— to you. When you eliminate them from your diet, you undergo withdrawal. The symptoms of withdrawal are unpleasant, regardless of how minor they actually may be, so your body craves the food. When you satisfy the craving, the symptoms disappear.

Few people have been taught to regard foods in this way, or to think of such a response as an "allergy." The common conception of food allergies involves itchy hives or, more seriously, such severe symptoms as one's throat swelling closed or even anaphylactic shock. Realign your thinking. Allergy to foods can and does cause symptoms of *all* kinds.

The next step is to identify the substances to which you may be allergic. Start with the one food or beverage you crave most and eliminate it from your diet for at least five days. Be extremely careful to ensure that the food in all its forms is eliminated totally. For example, if you constantly feel the urge to eat bread, make sure that there is no wheat in *anything* you eat. Check labels on all processed foods. Do not substitute pasta. The idea is to eliminate that food completely.

If you find your symptoms getting worse over the first three or four days, you can be fairly certain you are allergic to that food. The exacerbation of symptoms is a sign of withdrawal. By the fifth or sixth day, you should feel well. This may well be the time for you to see a clinical ecologist. What you will experience is similar to what has been outlined above; you will probably have to do a five-day fast again to clear your body of any possible residual effects from allergens. In addition, you will be asked to answer a wide range of questions which will help the doctor determine where to begin testing. These questions concern your sensitivities to all different foods, chemicals, and natural substances.

The testing may comprise one or more procedures. If the doctor is trying to determine which substances affect the patient, provocation testing (also called "clinical titration") will be conducted. There are different forms of this test: *sublingual,* in which the substance to be tested is placed under the tongue in the form of a dilute solution; *subcutaneous,* in which the solution is placed under the skin; *intracutaneous,* in which the substance solution is placed within the skin; and *nasal inhalation,* in which the substance is sprayed into the nose. Any and all responses to these tests are important, whether physical, perceptual, or mental. Even something as seemingly innocent as feeling sleepy or irritable has significance in this setting.

When the doctor wants to determine the comparative sensitivity a patient has to different substances (especially the common environmental substances we breathe daily), the "intracutaneous one-to-five serial dilution titration" is the test procedure used. In essence, the doctor performs a skin test using various strengths of solution (ranging from extremely diluted to only slightly diluted) prepared from the same excitant. The level of dilution at which skin-puffing or other symptoms occur indicates the severity of the patient's allergy—in other words, the more diluted the solution needed to provoke a reaction, the higher the degree of sensitivity indicated.

Neutralization of symptoms can be accomplished by introducing a diluted solution of the responsible substance. No one knows yet why this is, or how it works, but clinical ecologists have proven it so countless times. What has to be determined is what each patient's neutralizing dose is for each substance. Either of the two types of test mentioned above may be used. The need for this information is great; not all excitants can be avoided at all times. If the patient learns what the proper neutralizing dose is, he or she can keep a supply of that solution available to stop a reaction when it begins.

What is the real application of all this testing and theory for the sufferers of the various arthritic conditions? Unquestionably, symptoms can be, and have been, eased significantly by the elimination of certain foods and drinks from the patient's diets. Some clinical ecologists question whether all cases diagnosed as arthritis really are arthritis. There is evidence that in early cases the symptoms might be allergic symptoms and not the true disease. It is very possible that if the allergy is left untreated and the symptoms continue unabated, real damage will occur from the constant stress of the allergic symptoms. However, range of mobility, stiffness, pain, and even blood tests have shown improvement in many patients whose allergies have been relieved. There is no doubt that an individual in a milder stage of disease will benefit more than one in an advanced stage, simply because more damage has already occurred in the latter case. There is ample documentation that this system of testing and adjusting the patient's environment works and brings relief that is equal to medication therapy.

DIET

Many allergic reactions, including some of those that may be related to arthritic conditions, are associated with foods. What foods may be linked to arthritic symptoms? There is no single answer to that question. It is an individual problem for each patient, and has to be handled as such. However, the question leads us to an interesting area of treatment—diet. While diet is often a part of treatment as prescribed by allopathic doctors, there are also doctors trained in orthodox medicine who acknowledge that diet may, in fact, have some bearing on the symptoms of arthritis. Articles about this topic have been appearing in popular magazines as well.

AVOIDING NIGHTSHADE VEGETABLES

One subject under discussion is the effect of the nightshade family of vegetables on arthritis. There is evidence that these vegetables (tomatoes, eggplant, red pepper, and potatoes) somehow affect and exacerbate arthritis symptoms. Various alkaloids (scopalomine, nicotine, and atropine) that are present in these vegetables may be responsible for the adverse reactions that have been identified. In any event, many doctors do suggest that their arthritis patients avoid all these vegetables.

THE DONG DIET: AN EXAMPLE OF SUCCESS

One further extension of the dietary issue is a particular diet for arthritics. This diet was devised by Dr. Colin H. Dong, a graduate of Stanford University Medical School, in California, who was himself afflicted with arthritis. As he studied the available literature on the disease, and as his own illness progressively worsened, he became increasingly dissatisfied with the help available to him. The prospect of a lifetime of medication and the accompanying side effects displeased him. At one point, when his disease had become quite severe, he remembered a Chinese proverb that his father had repeated many times: "Sickness enters through the mouth and catastrophe comes out of the mouth."

The proverb inspired Dr. Dong to examine his diet, and the exercise had significant results. He had come far from the basic diet of rice, fish, and vegetables on which he had been raised. He decided to return to that way of eating, to eliminate all the processed foods, additives, high-fat foods, and so on that he had become accustomed to eating as an adult. To his relief, when he changed his diet the arthritis cleared; as he says, he had an almost complete remission from his crippling disease.

In light of the work done by the bio-ecologists, Dr. Dong's diet makes a great deal of sense. He eliminated foods that are frequently implicated as the source of allergy. Without those irritants in his system, his body was able to return to normal health.

This is not to say that all signs of a crippling form of arthritis or all the terrible symptoms of a rheumatic disease will melt away if one changes how one eats. But there is considerable evidence that for many people all the symptoms do disappear, and that for many other people a substantial degree of good health returns.

Dr. Dong's diet is fairly restrictive, and it reflects the times in which it was developed. For example, he does not allow egg yolk, or any whole-milk products. Until quite recently, cholesterol was known to be a cause of coronary heart disease, yet the mechanism of cholesterol metabolism and deposit was not fully understood. Patients were told that, to be safe, they should either eliminate or strictly limit cholesterol intake. More recent research has shown that cholesterol intake may not be related to cholesterol accumulation in the arteries. Thus, if one's cholesterol levels are not a problem, eggs and whole milk products can be taken safely. Although Dr. Dong's diet is sensible, provides a balance of the necessary nutrients, and can satisfy most people's dietary requirements, it should only be undertaken after consultation with a doctor.

The restrictions on the nightshade vegetables (see p. 52), and the diet devised by Dr. Dong are mentioned in this section on clinical ecology because both fit the general theory espoused by bio-ecologists. In light of evidence that some forms of rheumatic disease are autoimmune in nature, the concept of food allergies having an effect on one's condition makes even more sense. There is good reason to believe that as the body is continually subjected to allergens from foods, the immune system becomes overtaxed. Research may prove one day that just such an unrelenting burden is involved in the switch from a beneficial mechanism (which the immune system usually is) to a self-destructive one.

HOMEOPATHY

This system of health treatment was founded in the early 1800s by Samuel Hahnemann, a German physician. Homeopathy was a reaction against the prevaling medical practices, which involved blood-letting, purging, and other rather violent means of clearing the body of the ill "humors" (fluids), which were thought to cause illness. Hahnemann felt that these measures, along with the casual mixing of medicines that typified pharmacology of the period, did not constitute the correct manner of treating illness.

Hahnemann left the practice of medicine and became a translator of medical texts. It was while translating a work by a professor of medicine who claimed to have cured malaria by using cinchona bark (source of quinine) that Hahnemann began the studies that led to the development of homepathy. In brief, he did not agree with that professor's reason for the bark's curative powers, so Hahnemann tested the substance himself. He was able to bring on the symptoms of malaria by taking doses of the medication. What Hahnemann found out, and proved again many times with other medications, is that a medicine can reduce symptoms in a sick person yet, when given to a healthy person, that same medicine will produce the symptoms of the disease it is meant to cure.

Hahnemann was rediscovering a concept that had been expressed in the 10th century B.C. by the Hindus and again, in around 400 B.C., by Hippocrates, whose statement, "Through the like, disease is produced and through the application of the like, it is cured" had been repeated in the 16th century by Paracelsus, a famous Swiss doctor.

Hahnemann, interested in pharmacology, took the concept a

step further. He began testing the principle by experimenting with various natural drugs (the only kind available at the time) in order to determine just which medication caused which symptoms. In the course of his experiments, Hahnemann arrived at the now standard homeopathic practice of diluting the original material to a very mild potency.

According to homeopathic theory, the body is always working to keep itself in a balanced, or healthy, state. The term *vital force* is used to represent that balancing tendency. If the body is subjected to detrimental influences (e.g., germs or poisons), symptoms result. The symptoms have a definite part to play in the body's attempt to re-balance, or regain health. To a homeopath, symptoms are a good sign. The remedy prescribed to the patient is a supportive measure; it stimulates the "vital force" needing help at that time. It was Hahnemann's belief that only a very small amount of any drug would suffice to invigorate the "vital force," and therefore used highly diluted doses.

This system is quite different from allopathic medicine as practiced by most doctors today. The homeopathic physician is not as concerned with determining the exact cause of the illness or condition as he or she is with increasing the body's ability to become well again. To this end, the homeopathic doctor is very concerned with the *entire* patient, i.e., his or her physical and mental condition. Symptoms of both states are taken into account when choosing a remedy.

The most important part of a homeopathic doctor's job is to observe even the most minute details of a patient's condition. This involves asking a variety of questions that at first might seem unrelated to health. In keeping with the belief that the body comprises a system of interdependent parts, such a method of history-taking (called "taking the case" by homeopaths) makes sense. If one's emotions are affected by physical discomfort, for example, they can be as helpful an indicator of what treatment is needed as a physical complaint would be. As a result, the homeopathic physician spends a great deal of time with the patient in order to determine just what the "full picture" is. Only then can the doctor start to make an informed judgment as to which remedy will be most beneficial. What works for a patient with a flu-like set of symptoms one time may not help the next time. The nature of the illness may be different, and this difference can sometimes be shown by a seemingly unrelated symptom, such as whether the patient feels better in cool rooms than in hot ones.

For the treatment of a chronic condition or ailment, the doctor lists all the symptoms, makes special note of what are called the "strong" symptoms (those that are most pressing), and considers, too, what homeopaths call the "strange, rare, and peculiar" symptoms. These would include such things as the craving for, or aversion to, a particular food or drink. When the doctor has all that information, the next step is to consult the *Repertory of the Homeopathic Materia Medica,* which lists each of the "strong" symptoms and the drugs that cause them. For each of the patient's strong symptoms, the doctor notes the drugs indicated. After checking all of those strong symptoms, the doctor sees which one drug is the same for all or, if there is one drug that can cause all, which drug shows up most often. The doctor then refers back to the *Materia Medica* for a detailed description of each remedy, and double checks that the remedy chosen does, in fact, fit the symptoms noted. Then the treatment can begin.

This is what homeopaths call "constitutional prescribing." This is used for a condition that will not ease or disappear by itself. Sometimes one dose will be effective for a long period of time, as the proper remedy in such cases can spur the "vital force" dramatically.

One of the phenomena encountered in homeopathic treatment is called *aggravation*, which often occurs when the patient first starts the course of medication. Initially the symptoms may seem to worsen, and may last in that state for a day or two before general improvement is noticeable. This is a good sign, rather than one to cause concern. The premise is that a sick person is especially sensitive to the similar remedy, and so the symptoms will increase at first. The aggravation, therefore, shows that the proper remedy has been prescribed.

Homeopathic doctors try to prescribe as little medication as possible. Remedies are rarely mixed, and a person taking a constitutional remedy should not add another remedy without consulting his or her physician. When improvement is first noticed, the patient can take the remedy less frequently, with intervals between doses growing until improvement is certain. At that point, the patient should stop taking the remedy; too much will cause the symptoms to recur.

The nature of homeopathic medicine is such that there is no clear, single treatment for arthritis and related conditions. The choice of a remedy for a patient at any given time depends on a great number of variables; those variables may well differ among patients, and may even differ for a single patient at different times. Many homeopathic physicians believe that it is possible, however, with time and some effort on the patient's part, for a patient to become familiar with the remedies most often used and, if necessary, to prescribe his or her own remedy at a particular moment.

Certain remedies are recommended for acute conditions such as sprains and might, in fact, be among the choices a homeopathic doctor would make in treating arthritis. What you must remember is that homeopathy does not treat a "disease," if one defines the term as constituting a single, static condition. The symptoms are what matter, and homeopathy takes into account that symptoms constantly change.

CHIROPRACTIC

The system of chiropractic treatment as it is known today was developed near the end of the 19th century by Daniel David Palmer, in Davenport, Iowa. Although various manipulative methods and procedures have been used throughout history, by societies as diverse as ancient Greece, ancient Syria, the Aztecs, and ancient Japan, Palmer's method differed from these others. He was concerned exclusively with the vertebrae, the nervous system, and how the two affected the state of a person's health. In his effort to develop a systematic approach to health care and healing, Palmer eventually came to the conclusion that good health depends on channels of communication within the body remaining unobstructed. These channels, in his view, were the nerves.

Palmer believed that since impulses travel to and from the brain along nerves, and since the nerves pass through the vertebrae from the spinal column to all parts of the body, the position of the spinal column was of utmost importance. If even one vertebra were out of alignment, the pressure it would put on the nerves that pass through it could affect the body negatively.

As with many other forms of health treatment, Palmer's system of chiropractic had a name for the "force" that unifies the body and strives for a balanced, healthy, condition. Palmer called it *innate intelligence.* He understood that vertebrae could be misaligned as a result of an ancient or even a muscle contraction; even years of standing upright (for which the spine was not designed) could throw the spinal column out of line. Palmer stated that this pressure on the nerves causes irritation, excitation, and inflammation, all of which impeded the ability of the "innate intelligence" to convey information throughout the body.

In the nearly 100 years since Palmer set forth his ideas, the use of chiropractic has grown tremendously. Not surprisingly, the increasing knowledge about the body and its functioning has helped chiropractic evolve into a system that uses and benefits from that knowledge and from modern technology as well. In spite of this evolution, the basic component of treatment remains the same: the chiropractic *adjustment* of which so many people hear but may know nothing is, today, as Palmer developed it. The term used by chiropractors to describe what the adjustment consists of is *dynamic thrust.* This is a sudden and precisely placed force, applied to the vertebra that is misaligned. The displacement of a vertebra, so that the normal structural linking between that vertebra and those directly above and below it is no longer intact, is termed *subluxation.* As Palmer knew, with nerves branching out from the spinal column to the very extremities, a subluxation can elicit symptoms anywhere, not only at the point of displacement.

If you go to a chiropractor today for your arthritis, the doctor will make use of a variety of diagnostic tools. The most important of these is a detailed physical examination of the spine and the entire skeleton. This may include a postural analysis and mobility tests, to aid the chiropractor in assessing the full extent of your disease. X rays, blood tests, and even electrocardiograms, are now part of the diagnostic process. Although classical chiropractic did not have these tools, most chiropractors today feel that it is necessary to have as much information on hand as possible to help the patient; modern technology is not excluded. These tests help the chiropractor determine whether internal organs are affected and, if so, to what degree. The tests also serve as an indicator of how much function these organs and tissues can regain. Chiropractors are interested in the body's natural recuperative ability being permitted to function as it should; they accomplish this for the patient by removing the impediment (specifically the vertebra) from the nerves.

Chiropractors who treat arthritis know that there are different causes of the various conditions, but emphasis is placed on alleviating the stress and strain on the affected joint(s). Whether the damage to the joint developed from a trauma or from subluxations that, in turn, place strain on the nerves and organs or muscles affected by those nerves, the chiropractic adjustment will remove the irritation and help the patient both regain mobility and experience less pain.

It is generally accepted among chiropractors that treatment of subluxations can provide preventive care to a patient. If the body is in alignment and there is no, or at least reduced, internal strain, the chance is great that arthritis will not develop. In some cases of rheumatic disease, chiropractic treatment can stop its progress and can relieve pain as effectively as medication, without the latter's frequent harmful side effects. Though knowledge of nutrition (chiropractors are well trained in nutrition), and through what can be described as a "holistic" awareness of the patient, the chiropractor is able to counsel the arthritic to improve his or her entire physical and emotional state, all of which can only help in fighting the disease.

NATUROPATHY

Naturopathic medicine is a system of healing similar to homeopathy. Both rely on using natural substances in the healing process. Naturopathic medicine differs from homeopathy in many basic areas, however.

The philosophy behind this system is based on the concept of vital force, *vis medicatrix naturae,* which constitutes the body's power to heal itself and adapt to external environmental changes. All ministrations of a naturopathic physician are planned to stimulate and enhance this natural healing force. None of the therapeutic substances or procedures used interfere with this natural healing force.

As a holistic approach to health and healing, naturopathic medicine investigates possible hereditary, biological, emotional, and environmental problems. Disease is not considered a distinct, separate state of being; symptoms of disease are seen as being momentary, rather than chronic. In examining a patient, the naturopathic doctor discovers the various components of the illness. In this way the most fundamental cause can be determined, allowing for a treatment plan that eliminates the cause, which may be a nutritionally or environmentally caused imbalance.

Doctors of Naturopathy are trained in human anatomy, biochemistry, diagnostic techniques, herbal medications, homeopathy, acupuncture, physiotherapy, counseling, and many other natural procedures and therapies. There is no formal procedure as in allopathic medicine; naturopathic doctors develop their methods of treatment using those elements which they feel work best.

Practitioners of naturopathic medicine instruct patients in preventive methods. Naturopathic doctors teach patients how to return to good health—and stay there. This is as much a part of a naturopathic physician's practice as healing is.

Before a naturopathic doctor can treat a patient, he or she must first make a full assessment of that person's health. This is accomplished through a complete physical examination; a study of the patient's health history; and blood, urine, and often hair analyses. The patient's mental attitude, as well, gives the naturopath a better picture of the health profile.

The blood tests given are very thorough, revealing the condition of the blood itself and of the blood chemistry. Red blood cell counts, the amount of hemoglobin, white blood cell counts, and clotting time are all checked to determine whether: the body is producing enough of the various blood cells; there is infection (too many white blood cells would indicate that); the body is deficient in iron (reflected in the amount of hemoglobin); and clotting occurs normally. Insufficiency or abnormality of any of these factors is quite significant, and will provide the naturopathic physician with warning signs. The blood chemistry tests indicate the status of chemical functioning throughout the body. The various organs and glands produce and/or process different chemicals; if these are at abnormal levels either way, or even absent altogether, the naturopath can determine with greater certainty what the patient's condition is, and how to treat it.

Urine specimens provide information on several bodily functions. There may be too many waste products of metabolism (urea, uric acid, and creatinine levels show this); blood may be in the urine (which would indicate kidney or bladder disease or infection); the presence of glucose would indicate the need to check further for diabetes. Albumin (a protein) signifies that something is wrong somewhere in the body and needs to be researched. There may be bile pigments, which would point to a liver disorder. These findings, combined with those of the blood tests and the information from the patient's history, indicate how the body is working; if there are any disorders, the different readings will show where they are. These tests are standard medical tests, and are used by allopathic doctors as well as naturopathic, homeopathic, and osteopathic doctors.

Hair samples, too, can yield valuable information about the buildup of heavy metals in the system. Such elements as mercury and lead will be present in the hair if more than the normal trace amounts accumulate in the body. By measuring the quantity of these metals in the hair, the naturopath can evaluate the presence of a metal as a cause, or symptom, of any functional or chemical disorders.

Once the naturopath has all these data, a therapeutic program is planned for the patient's individual needs. Chinese medicine and acupuncture are among the treatment choices available; they work to re-balance the body's restorative powers. Homeopathy (see p. 53), another form of treatment in the naturopathic physician's repertoire, can be useful in relieving certain symptoms, bringing the patient back to a healthy state. Physical medicine plays a major role, with heat, light, water, sound, and electrical therapies to draw on. The lack of a balanced spectrum of light, for example, is known to cause depression and even physical symptoms in people.

The naturopath has a vast selection of treatment approaches

from which to choose. A given patient's program may combine a few, or several, of these treatments. So much depends on the patient's condition, past history, and the body of experience accumulated by not just the particular practitioner, but all naturopaths. Certainly one of the most vital aspects of any treatment is proper nutrition. The nutritional imbalances are best corrected in food, whenever possible; if not, vitamin and mineral supplements are used. The naturopath may choose to prescribe glandular extracts to compensate for poor functioning of the patient's own glands. The term "prescribe" is used in its literal sense here; none of the vitamins, minerals, or extracts requires a prescription. All may be bought at health food stores, at pharmacies, or from suppliers through the mail.

VITAMIN AND MINERAL SUPPLEMENTS

The various vitamins and minerals have been tested by doctors to help patients with arthritis, with some exciting results. Vitamin C, originally identified in the early 1930s by Dr. Albert Szent-Gyorgyi, has been used to alleviate osteoarthritis to a significant degree. This was reported in 1980 by Dr. James Greenwood, a doctor in Texas. Similar results had been reported in the *New England Journal of Medicine* a full 30 years before, in which the physician conducting the experiment stated that Vitamin C has definite antirheumatic properties when given in sufficiently high doses.

What is very important when following a therapeutic program of vitamin and mineral supplements is to have periodic blood and urine tests run as a check to show how well your body is using these supplements. Most of the vitamins and minerals are not dangerous in high doses, especially when the body is ill and, therefore, in need of greater amounts of those substances. Certain vitamins, however, can be toxic. No one really knows at what dosage any individual will react negatively; it is better to check and be certain you're making positive progress than to assume so and find out differently the hard way. Like allopathic regimens, naturopathic "prescriptions" should be followed carefully.

Aside from vitamin C, other vitamins have proven useful in treating and relieving many symptoms of different rheumatic diseases. Vitamin E is one. A study conducted in Israel, and reported in the July 1978 edition of *The Journal of The American Geriatrics Society,* tested vitamin E at a daily dosage of 600 International Units. The results of the study were very promising, and pointed to the viability of Vitamin E as an antirheumatic agent. Fully one-half of the subject patients enjoyed a "marked relief from pain" during the vitamin E portion of their participation.

Another vitamin that has been useful in treating arthritic conditions is niacinamide, one of the B vitamins. Empirical findings with his patients in the 1940s and 50s led Dr. William Kaufman, then in practice in Stamford, Connecticut, to a firm belief that niacinamide not only relieved pain but also had a definite, positive impact on ease of movement. His total patient population exceeded 650 arthritics. Dr. Kaufman's investigations with this vitamin were among the earliest; there are doctors throughout the country using it now.

It is important to note here that the doctors mentioned by name in this discussion are all M.D.s; that is, none is a naturopath. The reason these various studies are included in this section is that the mode of treatment coincides with that of naturopaths. It is highly significant (from a medical-politics point of view) that most of these doctors, and their work, are either disregarded or repudiated by most doctors who practice traditional allopathic medicine. The naturopathic and chiropractic communities have, on the other hand, responded positively to these and other studies and to the support these individual "orthodox" doctors have given to the nutritional movement.

B₆ is another of the B complexes that is used in treating rheumatoid and osteoarthritis. Dr. Robert Atkins, a New York doctor, prescribes it in high doses (up to 1,000 mg per day). Pantothenic acid, yet another B vitamin, was found to be at lower than normal levels in the blood of osteoarthritis patients in an English study. The degree of pain seemed related to the level of pantothenic acid, with greatest severity accompanying the lowest amounts. There is a significant correlation there, made more noteworthy by the researchers' findings that, when administered to patients over long periods of time, pantothenic acid was helpful in relieving symptoms. There is evidence, too, that many other B vitamins have their usefulness in treating different rheumatic conditions.

Vitamin D has advocates among the doctors who espouse nutritional therapy. It is necessary in the body; without it calcium is not absorbed and utilized to its fullest extent. Deficiency of this vitamin can cause rickets; the typically fragile bones of that disease are similar to the problem of weakening bones that afflicts many rheumatoid arthritis patients. The connection between the two conditions is significant, and in fact, therapeutic doses of vitamins A and D have proven beneficial to patients. Cod-liver oil seems the most directly useful form in which to take the vitamins.

Along with vitamins, minerals are necessary for the body's continued functioning. As with so many other substances, ingestion of minerals does not guarantee their full utilization. Absorption is the issue in question, and it is one that is not fully understood by doctors and scientists. Interactions between and among various materials may inhibit or enhance the amount absorbed of any of them. For example, chocolate blocks the absorption of calcium, and with vitamins A, D, and E, presence of all is necessary for the fullest use of any one.

Calcium is one of the most important minerals for arthritics. Although calcium deposits at joints can be a problem with certain forms of rheumatic conditions, more often than not patients with these diseases suffer from a calcium deficiency. The deposits occur after the body, desperate for calcium, draws it from the bones, leaving them weakened; the deposits are an attempt to "brace" the bones at the joints. Aging affects the body's need for, and ability to process, calcium. This ability lowers with age, while the need to process calcium increases. What many people do not realize is that even if one gets the government-suggested minimum daily requirement (800 mg), all of it is not always absorbed and used. Calcium works in concert with other elements: phosphorous, magnesium, vitamins D, A, and C, and hydrochloric acid (produced in the stomach). If the body is deficient in any of these, the others will not be assimilated properly, and thus none will be properly used in the body. Raising the intake of any one of these substances (with the exception of the stomach acid) means the rest have to be assessed and raised, too, to their proper complementary levels. Too many alkaline foods will neutralize the acid in the stomach; this, also, leads to poor utilization of minerals.

This discussion points out, again, the need to have these various minerals and vitamins evaluated periodically by a practitioner who can interpret test results properly and prescribe accordingly.

Sulfur is another mineral that is found concentrated in the joints. It has been used for centuries to ease some of the complaints of rheumatoid arthritis and osteoarthritis in the form of mineral baths, in which patients would immerse themselves. The actual therapeutic value of this mineral is becoming more clearly understood as research answers many questions about the impact of minerals on body functioning. Sulfur is supplied in the body by foods, specifically by three of the essential amino acids (found in dietary proteins): cysteine, histidine, and methionine. There have been reports connecting lowered levels of these amino acids with arthritic complaints; when doctors in both experimental and clinical situations increased the amounts of these amino acids, the rheumatic symptoms eased considerably.

Dr. Donald Gerber, a physician in New York, reported on the inability to metabolize copper in 50% of a group of arthritics he treated and studied. This rate was much higher than in a group of nonarthritics whom he had also studied. This finding seems significant and is bolstered by a report of studies conducted at the University of Cincinnati in the mid 1970s. The biochemists who were in charge of the experiments discovered that when combined with copper, aspirin was 30% more effective than cortisone in its ability to control inflammation. This was far superior to plain aspirin's effectiveness for the same purpose, rated at only 6% that of cortisone. All these studies point to the essential role that minerals play in treating the various rheumatic conditions. As with all the vitamins and minerals, it is necessary to increase the amount utilized by the body without reaching toxic levels. It may well be that with copper, food sources are more reliable than supplements. This is something your practitioner will know.

Other minerals that have been shown to play an important role in rheumatic disease include iodine, zinc, iron, manganese, and selenium; the list will probably grow as research becomes more focused on this promising aspect of disease prevention and control. If your naturopath recommends a vitamin or mineral program, question anything you do not understand or agree with; your understanding can only enhance the process. Always remember to follow the prescription of these supplements exactly. Do not skip doses, as the proper balance between and among the various substances must be maintained. Above all, make sure you get periodic check-ups and blood tests.

ACUPUNCTURE

Acupuncture is an ancient Chinese system of medical treatment that is based on the Chinese view of health and illness. As a treatment system, acupuncture is increasingly visible in the West; research during the past two decades has given stronger physical evidence to support the concepts of acupuncture, making it more acceptable to those with traditional scientific training.

The Chinese believe that good health exists when the life force, which they call *T'chi*, circulates freely through the body. Two opposing energies, *Yin* (negative) and *Yang* (positive), influence and control T'chi. The energy flows through *meridians* (of which there are 12). Stress (either actual illness or of the tension variety) can block this energy, with illness occurring or spreading as a result. Release of the pent-up energy allows the balance between Yin and Yang to return. Acupuncture is the process of releasing that energy. It involves the insertion of very fine needles into the skin at certain spots along the meridians. Proper choice of spots along the various meridians is based on a number of factors, all of which are integral to Chinese medicine. They include the different pulses (there are six in all, three superficial and three deep), a knowledge and understanding of the five elements (wood, fire, earth, metal, and water), and an understanding of the principles of Yin and Yang. These last two, representing the masculine (negative) and feminine (positive) forces of nature respectively, are associated with particular organs of the body, the Yin organs being solid and the Yang organs being hollow. Each Yin organ has its corresponding Yang organ, and each pair has corresponding tissues associated with it. The forces of Yin and Yang are stored in special areas called burning spaces; from these, Yin and Yang travel throughout the body along the meridians.

The greatest objection to acupuncture among orthodox medical physicians has been the lack of scientific evidence of structures— meridians, a network linking the insertion spots (and these spots are *not* random, they are quite specific). But research by Soviet doctors has proven that the density of skin at acupuncture sites (whether acupuncture had ever been performed or not) was less than the density of skin at other places on the body. Similarly, two Soviet scientists discovered that the skin's temperature was different at acupuncture sites from the temperature elsewhere on the skin.

In 1963, a Korean doctor announced findings concerning electrical resistance in the skin. His research showed that tracings of the variations of the skin's electrical resistance corresponded perfectly with the drawings of the acupuncture meridians from a 5,000 year old textbook of Chinese medicine. Another significant finding of his research was that the structure of other skin cells along the meridians differed from the structure of other skin cells, and most importantly, that at the acupuncture points themselves, there occurred small groupings of an unusual type of cell.

Sir Henry Head, an English doctor who was alive in the late 1800s, isolated certain areas of the skin that were affected by certain specific illnesses. These areas came to be called "Head's zones" and were the basis for a German-developed treatment procedure called *Heilanasthesie* (therapeutic anesthesia). By deadening particular areas of skin, doctors were able to alleviate pain in corresponding organs. Taking the concept one step further, doctors have found that injections of local anesthesia at specific Head's zones will both relieve pain and, in many cases, aid in curing the underlying disease.

These, then, are among the scientific reports that have given credence to acupuncture. Increasingly, acupuncture is being used to relieve chronic pain, and has been found to be more effective than steroids with none of the side effects. It is interesting to note that the procedure is accepted much more widely in Europe than in the United States.

So far as rheumatic disease is concerned, the use of acupuncture has its greatest demonstrated value to date in easing chronic pain. Many of the pain management clinics—which are becoming an increasingly important part of the American health care system—rely on acupuncture as one of the forms of treatment employed to help patients learn to live with their conditions. There is strong evidence that, for at least the early stages of certain of the rheumatic diseases, or for some mild forms of these diseases, acupuncture can be of value in reversing the course of the disease. Inflammation in localized conditions can be eased substantially by acupuncture, and doctors now are expanding the application of this procedure to fight inflammation in more damaging conditions.

ALTERNATIVE TREATMENT

Medications	Surgery	Exercise	Diet	Note
CLINICAL ECOLOGY				
In serious cases, may need to remain on some of the medications listed under ORTHODOX MEDICINE AND OSTEOPATHY, but dosage may be reduced.	See note*	Specific exercises may be used.	Specific rotation diet	Clinical Ecology does not claim a cure, but can often reduce symptoms enough to prevent the need for surgery or drugs.
DIET				
See note*	See note*	See note*	Highly restrictive diet	Patients using diet generally follow the same guidelines as those used by patients of Clinical Ecologists.
HOMEOPATHY				
Drugs prescribed based on symptoms, as indicated in the *Repertory of Homeopathic Materia Medica.* As little medication given as possible; medications mixed rarely	See note*	See note*	See note*	Each homeopathic physician has his own view as to other treatment.

CHIROPRACTIC	Not licensed to practice surgery	Not permitted to prescribe but often will work in conjunction with M.D.s who can. Vitamins, minerals, and glandular extracts often used	See note*	Chiropractors are highly trained in nutrition and will often modify patient's diet to try to ease symptoms.	Emphasis placed on alleviating the stress on afflicted joints through physical adjustments. An exercise program may be prescribed.
NATUROPATHY	See note*	Herbal remedies and vitamins, minerals, and glandular extracts	Specific exercises may be used.	Naturopaths are highly trained in nutrition, and will often modify patient's diet to try to ease symptoms.	Acupuncture used extensively, as well as heat, water, sound, and electrical therapies

* The treatment guidelines for the following approaches to arthritis are holistic in nature; therefore no differentiations are made for the various forms of arthritis.

5

RESEARCH

RESEARCH INTO THE CAUSES OF RHEUMATIC DISEASE

There is no consensus on the cause of arthritis—it seems to have a number of different causes. Through research and experimentation, the medical community has gained an increasing understanding of many of these. What follows is a summation of important research in this area.

Cartilage structure and metabolism   It is now known that enzymes (collagenase is one) can erode cartilage. Study continues, particularly in an attempt to relate enzyme release to biomechanical forces. This is especially important in countering the development of osteoarthritis.

Inflammation   Although the inflammatory processes that damage joint structures in rheumatoid arthritis are better understood now than ever before, research to determine which substances influence those processes is still under way. The role of prostaglandins in the release of erosive enzymes is not yet fully understood and is one of the areas that promises important advances in the treatment of synovitis.

The immune system   The workings of the immune system are just beginning to unfold. Researchers have made progress in understanding the role of immune complexes produced by this system, the regulation of immune reactions, and the inflammation and other tissue destruction that occur when the immune system breaks down or becomes misdirected.

Epidemiology and genetics   The identification of genetic markers in various rheumatic diseases has provided an important diagnostic and pre-diagnostic tool. Research is being conducted to investigate the possibility and probability that other rheumatic diseases are linked to similar markers.

Infectious triggers Lyme arthritis (p. 9), which was first identified in 1976, was eventually discovered to have been caused by a tick bite. This disease now serves as a model for the study of infection as an initiator of arthritis, and for the study of treating such a form of arthritis.

NATIONAL INSTITUTE OF ARTHRITIS, DIABETES, AND DIGESTIVE AND KIDNEY DISEASES (NIADDK)

The National Institute of Arthritis, Diabetes, and Digestive and Kidney Diseases (p. 126) hereinafter referred to as NIADDK, is the single most important center of research into the different rheumatic diseases in the United States. It supports research at universities, hospitals, and medical schools across the country and has an active research program of its own conducted by its Arthritis and Rheumatism branch. The branch's studies are carried out at the Warren G. Magnuson Clinical Center, which is part of the National Institutes of Health (NIH).

Although NIH comprises federally funded institutions of "orthodox" medicine, the approaches of the research programs are wide ranging. Areas of investigation have included new drugs, the uses of vitamins and their derivatives, the nature of autoimmune responses, the role of allergies in rheumatic conditions, and new surgical techniques. The list is far longer, and is best discussed in terms of each separate disease.

RESEARCH INTO SPECIFIC FORMS OF ARTHRITIS

RHEUMATOID ARTHRITIS

NIADDK supports numerous investigations in the search for better drug therapy for rheumatoid arthritis. One such program, at the Dartmouth-Hitchcock Multipurpose Arthritis Center (New Hampshire) under the direction of Dr. Edward D. Harris, Jr., is testing the effects of two forms of retinoic acid on the synovial lining cells of patients with RA. This is a significant investigation because retinoic acid is a vitamin A derivative; success would imply that vitamins may be useful in other forms than just supplements. In fact, the results of these particular studies show that these drugs completely inhibit the production of collagenase (an enzyme that destroys joint cartilage), and moderately reduce levels of prostaglandin E_2 (a fatty acid that both contributes to inflammation and slows the formation of new cartilage). The positive effects of retinoic acid are quite similar to those of the steroids (p. 31), yet preliminary results show little of the undesirable side effects of the steroids.

The discovery of the steroid methylprednisolone (p. 33) was made by Dr. Henry Lee who, with his colleagues at the Florida A&M School of Pharmacy, worked under a grant from NIADDK. This was a significant advance, for tests with laboratory animals indicated that this new compound had the beneficial effects of its "parent" drug, prednisolone, without the damaging effect that drug has on the adrenal system.

Work is continuing on a new experimental form of treatment for rheumatoid arthritis: radiation of lymph glands and other lymphoid tissues. "Total lymphoid irradiation" (TLI) tends to suppress the immune system; it has been an effective and safe treatment for Hodgkin's disease for 20 years. Scientists, therefore, have reasoned that it might improve the symptoms of autoimmune diseases. Dr. David Trentham, at the Multipurpose Arthritis Center at Brigham and Women's Hospital in Boston, used this technique to treat 10 patients with severe rheumatoid arthritis. He found that TLI significantly reduced joint inflammation in several of the patients for at least six months, with no serious side effects from the radiotherapy. These results point to the advisability of further investigations into how long TLI's effectiveness lasts and whether studies continue to show a lack of side effects. What may prove to be the most important result of this work concerns the role of T cells, a type of white blood cell, in immuno-inflammation. This may lead to other treatments that specifically correct T cell dysfunction.

One of the more serious complications of longstanding rheumatoid arthritis is inflammation of the blood vessels, called vasculitis. This can become a life-threatening condition. Research conducted by Dr. John Davis at the University of Virginia School of Medicine showed that rheumatoid vasculitis can be successfully treated with cyclophosphamide (p. 38), one of the immunosuppressive drugs. As the condition of patients on this treatment improves, the level of immune complexes in their blood decreases. These complexes are combinations of antibodies and antigens; the correlation noted above suggests that these immune complexes have a role in the blood vessel inflammation that occurs in rheumatoid arthritis.

OSTEOARTHRITIS

Biomechanical studies measure and model the mechanical forces, geometry, and lubrication of normal and diseased joints. Several NIADDK-supported investigators are working on the challenging and complex task of developing devices that can measure forces from within the joints themselves. Dr. Thomas Brown at the University of Pittsburgh is investigating the use of wafer-thin pressure transducers to be inserted into knee joints. At Case Western Reserve University (Cleveland, Ohio), Drs. R.H. Brown, K.G. Heiple, and V.M. Goldberg are creating joint replacements that contain tiny instruments to measure forces on the joints. These doctors have just recently been able to use an instrumented hip replacement on a patient volunteer, which should yield valuable information. The same group is working on an instrumented knee replacement.

One new project involves using grafts from an individual's rib tissue to induce cartilage growth on the ends of bones that form joints. This work, conducted by Dr. Richard Coutts at the University of California, San Francisco, follows earlier experiments in which this technique was used successfully in human finger joints. It is hoped that the technique will be applicable to the knee and other large joints.

Animal studies make possible investigation of theories and techniques that are not ready for trial on humans. In one such set of studies, under the direction of Dr. Carl Brighton at the University of Pennsylvania, cartilage is being retrieved, preserved, and transplanted to joints. Dr. Brighton's purpose is to determine the biochemical and biomechanical properties of such tissue. This information will help doctors identify possible barriers to this technique and will point to problems that must be overcome before the technique can be tested in patient volunteers.

JUVENILE RHEUMATOID ARTHRITIS

One important area of research in the attempt to better understand juvenile rheumatoid arthritis is concerned with identifying genetic markers, factors present in people with an inherited tendency toward a disease. This research might enable physicians to determine which children are at risk for some form of JRA and promptly diagnose and treat those with JRA, so that complications could be prevented or minimized.

Dr. Peter Schur and his colleagues at Brigham and Women's Hospital in Boston have found an increased frequency of the marker LHA-DRw5 in children with a form of JRA that carries a particular risk of iritis. This finding shows that this form of JRA may be inherited; it may also help predict which children with JRA are likely to develop this eye complication.

At Johns Hopkins University, in Baltimore, at the Multipurpose Arthritis Center, Drs. Thomas Zizic and Mary Betty Stevens have been studying genetic markers. They found the marker HLA-B27 (previously identified in patients with other forms of rheumatic disease) in patients with a rare form of JRA; these patients were young women who in childhood had developed a form of arthritis that, while initially similar to rheumatoid arthritis, progresses to an unusual form of spondylitis that can lead to fusion of the neck vertebrae in addition to inflammation of the joints.

SYSTEMIC LUPUS ERYTHEMATOSUS

Much of the current research on lupus focuses on the immune system and the role of antigens (substances that provoke the immune response) and antibodies (substances that are produced by the body to destroy the antigens). Lupus experiments have been carried out in specially developed strains of mice. Studies of these mice and of patients with lupus have demonstrated that certain types of white blood cells that normally keep the antibody-producing cells in check are defective when lupus is present. These observations have been confirmed by teams of investigators, including Dr. Peter Schur of Brigham and Women's Hospital, Boston, and Dr. Alfred Steinberg of NIADDK's Arthritis and Rheumatism branch. The teams have also found that decreases in these white cells were clearly correlated with disease activity. Replacement of the deficient cell material may be a possible treatment for lupus in future years.

Dr. Schur and his associates have also been investigating several immunologic antigen-antibody reaction tests in an effort to improve the effectiveness of the methods used to diagnose and treat lupus. They have found that abnormal levels of certain complement proteins and anti-DNA antibodies can predict when SLE may become active; this would guide the treatment of individual patients, and is a significant advance.

The importance of sex hormones in lupus has been established by various studies. Recently reported investigations at Rockefeller University, in New York, have identified a connection between lupus and estrogen. Women with lupus were found to have abnormal estrogen metabolism, a finding that points to the need for more studies in this area. At the University of California, San Francisco, Dr. Norman Talal and his associates have shown that estrogens accelerate SLE in mice, while androgens (male hormones) suppress the disease in mice. This study, too, indicates a need for further investigation in this area.

Dosages of various drugs can affect the course of treatment. Dr. Charles Christian, working at the Hospital for Special Surgery in New York, found that methylprednisolone (p. 33) has different effects at high doses than at low doses. Specifically, when given in pulses of high doses, this steroid can increase kidney function in lupus patients (disfunction of this organ is frequently a problem in SLE cases), improve clinical symptoms, and reduce the number of immune complexes in the blood, with fewer side effects than occur when lower, more continuous doses are given.

Drs. Zizic and Stevens (p. 69), in their work on genetic markers, have been able to identify factors that indicate which patients are at high risk for ischemic bone necrosis. This condition, in which the blood—and therefore oxygen—supply to bones is diminished, leading to bone deterioration, can be a serious problem. These doctors have also developed methods of early detection and treatment, based on identifying the factors mentioned above.

CLINICAL RESEARCH

Another very important part of the overall research program is clinical research.

NIADDK funds clinical studies at various institutions, including a consortium of 11 clinics that use common research protocols. This group is known as the Cooperative Systemic Studies in the Rheumatic Diseases, and the various component clinics are coordinated by a center at the University of Utah. The particular approach of this program allows in-depth research on a wide variety of rheumatic conditions. Some of the investigations by this group include long-term studies of the use of D-penicillamine (p. 34), oral gold salts (p. 33), and methotrexate in rheumatoid arthritis; the effectiveness of DMSO (p. 75) in treating the skin ulcers of scleroderma; and new studies on polyarteritis (inflammatory disease of the blood vessels, associated with certain rheumatic diseases) and polymyalgia rheumatica. The consortium keeps a patient registry and so has data on more than 7,500 patients.

The use of whole body CAT scans, which involves computer

assisted, three-dimensional X rays, is being studied as a substitute for bone biopsies to monitor mineral loss or replacement in bones of patients taking steroids (p. 31) for rheumatic diseases. If this process proves sufficiently accurate, it will mark a wonderful advance, eliminating the need for the surgical procedure, which always carries some risk.

One research goal has been the stimulation of bone growth by electrical currents. This technique originated as a method of treating fractures that would not heal easily; its applications could be broadened to other areas. At the University of Pennsylvania, in Philadelphia, Dr. Carl Brighton is studying the stimulation of bone growth in osteoporosis. Another investigation into the use of electrical stimulation involves a technique to enhance the fixation of artificial joints.

REPLACEMENT JOINTS

The need to perfect and improve currently available joint replacements and replacement techniques is the focus of much research. At the University of California, Los Angeles (UCLA), Dr. Harlan Amstutz is studying fixatives that would replace the cement now being used. Various substances are being tested to see which work best to encourage bone growth into the new joint. A new knee that has been devised, using a cobalt/chrome alloy, has yielded promising results in the early stages of investigation (p. 44). At the University of South Carolina, Dr. Myron Specter has been able to demonstrate good shear strength coupled with an early ingrowth of bone with porous plastic-coated prostheses. Another report states that greater strength of replacement joints can be achieved by precoating the stem of the prosthesis with cement. This investigation, conducted by Dr. Andreas Von Recum at Clemson University in South Carolina, found that not only was the new joint stronger when the stem was precoated, but surgery itself was simpler in these cases.

Joint strength is an important area of concern to patients. By determining when joints are loosening, doctors will be able to treat their patients more appropriately and to evaluate the various prostheses and surgical techniques more accurately. In turn, data on the various replacement joints and techniques will lead to better results.

To aid that effort, a sound emission testing device was recently developed by Dr. Timothy Wright and his colleagues at the Hospital for Special Surgery in New York. This device enables doctors to detect the loosening of artificial joints early; preliminary tests with it have detected clear differences between well-fixed hip replacements and those that were loose.

GOVERNMENT AGENCIES

Government agencies other than NIADDK are involved in studies that relate, either directly, or by extension, to the treatment of arthritis. At the National Cancer Institute (NCI), numerous questions concerning the immune system are being investigated: how it works, how it breaks down, why it breaks down, and so on. The results of these studies are as applicable to lupus and rheumatoid arthritis as they are to cancer. In one project, blood tests from rheumatoid arthritis patients showed an abnormally low count of a certain type of T cells. In addition, analysis of joint fluids from these patients showed that another type of T cell, normally found at a site of inflammation not due to chronic disease, was missing.

One of the other projects involved mice that developed SLE. These mice received injections of prostaglandin E1. This substance, produced in the human body, was able to prolong survival in the mice. It seems that the prostaglandin reduces the number of antigen-antibody complexes in specific parts of the kidneys. In autoimmune diseases such as SLE, these antigen-antibody complexes gather in the kidneys and prevent them from filtering body wastes efficiently. Prostaglandin E1 also seemed to cause a decrease in the amount of those complexes circulating in the blood. What is especially significant is that the prostaglandin did not suppress the normal functioning of the immune system. These findings point to the possibility that prostaglandin E1 may be clinically useful in treating SLE.

The National Heart, Lung, and Blood Institute (NHLBI) is interested in rheumatoid conditions because they may attack the heart, lungs, and blood vessels as well as joints.

The lungs may be affected in some cases of rheumatoid arthritis, and they are also vulnerable to certain of the collagen disorders. The vulnerability is understandable if one knows that connective tissue makes up more than 25% of total lung mass. The complications in the lungs from these diseases range from pleurisy (inflammation of the membrane that surrounds the lungs) to collapse of the lung(s), with almost every possible condition in between those extremes. The blood vessels and the heart are subject to inflammation, weakening, accumulation of blood clots, and blood deprivation due to ruptured or blocked blood vessels.

The NHLBI research programs are oriented primarily toward cardiopulmonary manifestations of rheumatoid diseases, but some studies concern the immunological aspects of these disorders. These studies treat some of the same problems that are considered vital by NIADDK and NCI, including immune system response and mechanisms, inflammatory cells and their workings, and the interrelationship between the immune system and inflammation. An advance in any one of these areas is of value to the research on the others, and reports of findings in any project at any of these institutes are of use to researchers working on related projects at the other institutes.

The National Institute of Dental Research (NIDR) also conducts and supports basic and applied research related to arthritis because of the shared nature of some major dental problems and diseases of joints. NIDR research projects related to arthritis fall, for the most part, into one of six categories: chemistry and molecular biology of connective tissue proteins and glycoproteins; abnormal and normal mechanisms of mineralization; craniofacial anomalies; temporomandibular joint disorders (this joint, called TMJ for short, is the hinge of the lower jaw where it joins the skull); periodontal diseases; and biomaterials.

Investigators in the NIDR Laboratory of Microbiology and Immunology are studying hormone-like substances secreted by wandering cells called macrophages and skin cells known as keratinocytes; these substances may be responsible for some of the joint inflammation that occurs in cases of scleroderma and rheumatoid arthritis. These researchers had already shown that macrophages produce Interleukin 1, a hormone-like substance that stimulates lymphocytes to produce antibodies. Interleukin 1 also activates synovial cells that trigger inflammatory processes within arthritic joints. Recent studies suggest that Interleukin 1 is produced by skin cells, too. These studies raise the possibility that Interleukin 1 may be a crucial factor in regulating inflammatory cell activity in rheumatoid arthritis, scleroderma, and dermatomyositis.

The development of non-poisonous, strong biomaterials is another area of interest. These biomaterials, which are being developed as dental implants, may also prove useful for joint replacements in arthritic patients. Dr. Allan Weinstein at Tulane University has compared the performance of three different implants placed in dogs' legs. Each of the implants is a new material; the success of the materials was measured by the radiographic appearance of the implant and by the amount of thickening of the outer layer of bone around the implant. The studies showed that two of the implants, one made of cobalt-chromium-molybdenum, the other of the same materials coated with bioglass, produced the greatest amount of bone thickening. Studies are continuing, with hopes that a usable substance will be the final result of all the work.

Increased knowledge of the factors that regulate bone formation and mineralization will be useful for the design of a sensible therapeutic approach to skeletal disorders such as osteoporosis. Within NIDR is the Laboratory of Biological Structure; Dr. A. Haridara Reddi leads a team that is investigating the role of factors associated with the protein matrix in regulating bone cell differentiation. Collagen is the prime component in this matrix, and is the chief protein in connective tissue. It is secreted by cells, forming a network (the matrix referred to above) between and around those cells. If demineralized bone matrix is implanted beneath the skin, new cartilage, bone, and bone marrow differentiation occurs at the site. This development is sequential, and proceeds in a defined and predictable schedule. The implant serves as a framework for cells to attach, multiply, and differentiate into bone cells. The study currently in progress is focused on further purification of extracellular matrix components, which have a part in spurring new bone growth. Recently, surgeons at Harvard Medical School and at UCLA Medical School have applied the technique of induced bone formation to correct skeletal and craniofacial defects. It is likely that this technique could also be used to strengthen bones that have been weakened by rheumatic diseases.

The National Institute of Allergy and Infectious Diseases (NIAID) is, like its sister institutes, conducting research that has applications to the rheumatic diseases. These studies focus on normal and abnormal functions of the immune system, mediators of inflammation, and immunogenic disease association.

One study, conducted by Dr. John R. David of Brigham and

Women's Hospital in Boston, is investigating cellular immunity. During earlier stages of this investigation, he was able to purify migration inhibitory factor, which is an important agent in an interaction between two types of white blood cells, T lymphocytes (T cells) and macrophages, that leads to cell mediated immune reactions and delayed hypersensitivity. Macrophages are a causative factor in cellular tissue inflammation.

Many of the arthritis-related diseases stem from pathologic changes in collagen, a main supportive protein of tendon, bone, cartilage, and connective tissue. Dr. David and his colleagues also studied collagen as an immune reactant, with the intention of learning how they might develop an animal model of autoimmunity. They found that, by binding spleen cells from a rat to its own collagen, then injecting the linked cells into the same rat, they could suppress induction of immune reactions against the collagen. These efforts are expected to help determine whether suppression of autoimmune phenomena might be beneficial to human arthritis or collagen disorders.

At the Asthma and Allergic Disease Center at the University of Kansas Medical School, a study is under way to determine the most effective route of administration for prednisolone (p. 33). Preliminary results of the study, which is headed up by Dr. Daniel Stechschulte, show daily oral doses to be more effective than intravenous pulse therapy ("pulse" refers to the timing of the doses) in their control of such clinical signs as sedimentation rate, blood count, and creatinine clearance. This same team is conducting studies to investigate the relationship between antibodies and suppressor T lymphocytes in SLE.

NIAID is supporting investigations, led by Dr. Ira Green, that have found that patients with SLE lack suppressor T cells, which may explain the increased levels of autoantibodies in these patients. There are far-reaching implications in Dr. Green's observation that plasma from patients with active SLE can induce defects in suppressor T cells of normal individuals.

Plasmapheresis (p. 40) has been investigated by Dr. Raphael J. De Horatius of Thomas Jefferson University in Philadelphia. He used the technique to remove circulating immune complexes from the blood in order to study the effect of such removal on immune regulation in SLE. His results disagree with those of Dr. Allen Kaplan, another NIAID grantee, who found in his studies that plasmapheresis could be beneficial. This discrepancy points to the need for further studies on this particular aspect of SLE and its treatment.

The National Institute of General Medical Sciences (NIGMS) supports research in basic biomedical fields, and many of these projects have applications to the treatment of rheumatic diseases. One such study, conducted by Dr. Robert M. Rose at the Massachusetts Institute of Technology, is designed to find ways to improve the wear characteristics of polythylene, used in joint replacements. Dr. A. Seth Greenwald, at the Cleveland Research Institute, is working with an implant material that is coated with a porous substance designed to allow new bone growth into the implant.

This would hold it in place more firmly than if it were cemented; a similar knee joint (p. 44) has already been tested in Baltimore.

The advances in research enable doctors to refine and redefine the diagnosis and treatment of rheumatic disease all the time. Patients reading about particular advances should realize that, for the most part, the research projects do not offer firm answers and/or treatments. Rather, they point the way for further study, leading to new and more certain progress.

There are situations in which experimental programs might be of value to a given patient. The National Institutes of Health do accept patients for inclusion in some of their studies; acceptance comes only after referral by a doctor and rigorous scrutiny of the patient's records. A patient may be called to Bethesda for preliminary examinations and/or testing to determine whether that person is right for the project under way. If you are chosen for such a project, all treatment is free of charge, as is the cost for the stay at Warren G. Magnuson Clinical Center, where the studies take place.

PRIVATE SECTOR RESEARCH

There are other centers of research than the government-sponsored institutes already mentioned. Most of the research conducted in universities, hospitals, and medical centers *is* funded through the government, but private, non-profit organizations sometimes provide monies for experimentation. Drug companies often do extensive research, but that is usually related to the use of a particular drug or group of drugs. Some very significant work and results derive from involvement of the private sector.

DMSO

One such project, which began in private industry and has since elicited government attention, is DMSO. This is a drug (dimethyl sulfoxide) whose use is quite controversial. It is a rather simple organic compound that occurs naturally; its two post-metabolized forms are normally present in man. It has been used as an industrial solvent for a long time, and the first reports on its pharmacological applications and therapeutic value appeared in 1964. The compound has several unusual attributes, most distinctive of which is its ability to permeate the skin, carrying with it other chemical compounds for absorption into the circulating blood within minutes of its application.

This strange capacity, as well as several others identified in laboratory experiments on animals, have definite implications for medical use. Aside from being able to penetrate intact membranes, DMSO can be used as an anti-inflammatory, a bacteriostatic agent, a local analgesic, a collagen solvent, a vasodilator (dilates blood vessels), a diuretic, and a cryoprotective agent (protects against damage from freezing). Studies on human patients have been conducted, also (some 100,000 patients had received DMSO by the end of 1965, according to a report by the National Academy of Science). These clinical trials showed the drug to be useful in treating a wide variety of conditions, including rheumatoid arthritis, gout, ankylosing spondylitis, and the skin manifestations of scleroderma.

Some critics of the drug pointed to the animal studies in which the lens in the eyes of test subjects underwent reversible changes. Thought to be related to DMSO, these changes had not been observed in a single human. Still, the clinical trials with the drug were stopped, although testing for possible toxicity in human eyes continued. As of 1980, no damage had been noted, so the U.S. Food and Drug Administration (FDA) lifted its ban on DMSO clinical trials.

The National Academy of Science (NAS) was asked to conduct an independent review of all available information on DMSO. Although both FDA and NAS felt that many of the early DMSO studies were poorly controlled, NAS concluded that the drug could be very effective in the treatment of certain conditions. The report of the NAS ad hoc committee states: "The reported clinical efficacy of DMSO in scleroderma . . . is such that investigation of its use under [this and other] circumstances should be pursued. . . . With respect to scleroderma . . . the conclusion has been reached on the grounds that, in view of the paucity of therapeutic resources of [this condition], any promising lead should be followed." It went on to say also that "There is suggestive evidence that DMSO may be effective . . . in relieving the pain of rheumatoid arthritis." The report confirmed that, other than the observed reversible eye problems in laboratory animals, the toxic effects of DMSO are few.

The political situation regarding DMSO is quite complicated; although the FDA has been rather reluctant to grant a New Drug Application for the drug for use in treating scleroderma (p. 8), certain states have legislated approval of DMSO for sale under certain conditions. Some states' medical societies have specifically opposed DMSO while others have favored and lobbied for its legalization. The availability of industrial and veterinary forms of DMSO further confuses the issue, as neither of these has a clear cut record of testing or proper application.

Beyond all the confusion surrounding DMSO—its legal status and available formulations—it remains true that untold numbers of people have found relief from their rheumatic conditions by using DMSO. The drug is usually applied topically at the site of inflammation, with relief reported to be almost immediate in many cases, and within minutes in the rest. Granted, of course, the relief is of a temporary nature. Experiments conducted prior to the ban in 1965 and since 1980 indicate that DMSO is useful in acute situations (which points to its efficacy in bursitis and tendinitis) rather than chronic conditions, to help soft tissue damage.

In scleroderma, collagen accumulates, blocking blood flow, thus creating skin ulcers. DMSO is able to dissolve the collagen, giving ulcers an opportunity to heal. The use of DMSO in sclerodermal ulcerations is being studied by the government, with approval likely if no toxicity is reported.

Criticism against DMSO has been leveled on several counts. One problem, according to critics, is that, with DMSO available in various non-controlled formulations, people can treat themselves and may harm themselves. There is no guarantee that any particular form of DMSO is pure; since it is absorbed into the system so easily it will carry any impurities into the bloodstream with it. Furthermore, when DMSO is used successfully to ease the discomforts of acute localized trauma, the patient may well end up overusing the injured area, or using it too soon, thus causing further damage. Another purported danger of DMSO is its enhancement of other drugs' actions. The hazard here is possible toxicity from another drug, as there is no way to predict to what degree those actions will be amplified.

The direct side effects encountered by test patients are relatively minor. A characteristic garlic-like taste in the mouth appears shortly after the DMSO is absorbed and lasts for several hours. Skin irritation and/or slight chemical burns at the point of application are the most common problems (although not widespread), and are more likely if the concentration of DMSO is a high one. Itching and welts at the site are next most common reactions, and there can be such symptoms as headaches, drowsiness, and nausea (with or without diarrhea).

The federal government and Research Industries Corporation (the manufacturer of government-approved DMSO for therapeutic use in interstitial cystitis) are involved in several research studies concerning DMSO. The trials relevant to rheumatic diseases are for: soft tissue trauma, rheumatoid arthritis, and scleroderma (at the Cooperative Systemic Studies in the Rheumatic Diseases, p. 70). During the next few years, reports of these various projects should be available, with information that will determine whether the promise of DMSO can be fulfilled.

6

HEALTH PROFESSIONALS, HOSPITALS, AND CLINICS

HEALTH PROFESSIONALS, HOSPITALS, AND CLINICS

This chapter contains information about individual health professionals, hospitals, and clinics that treat various rheumatic diseases.

Most of the individual practitioners who have entries were trained in, and practice, orthodox medicine. The reason for the absence of practitioners of such forms of treatment as chiropractic, homeopathy, and osteopathy is that these individuals usually regard themselves as holistic in outlook and treatment and therefore do not consider their practices to be focused specifically on the rheumatic diseases. Names of individual practitioners can be obtained from the national organizations, or registries, of the various schools of treatment (see Chapter 5, *Foundations, Organizations, and Self-Help Groups*, and Chapter 6, *Professional Societies*).

The hospitals and clinics listed here either treat arthritis directly, or treat the chronic pain that results from rheumatic conditions. It is important to note that almost every major teaching hospital in the country has a department of rheumatology and/or a specific arthritis clinic. Many are now developing pain control or management clinics as well.

Most of the information in this directory was gleaned from questionnaires completed by the individual practitioners, clinics, hospitals, or organizations. Some entrants have been included though their questionnaires were not returned, because their reputations warranted such inclusion. These entries are, by necessity, less complete than the others.

Preceding the A to Z listings, readers will find a handy list dividing the entries under the following headings: Traditional, Innovative, and Alternative.

Inclusion in this directory does not represent an endorsement or recommendation by either the editors or the publisher.

HEALTH PROFESSIONALS

TRADITIONAL

Alfred I. Dupont Institute
Roy D. Altman, M.D.
Harlan Amstutz, M.D.
Arthritis and Back Pain
   Center, Inc.
Peter Barland, M.D.
John Baum, M.D.
J. Claude Bennet, M.D.
Sheldon Blau, M.D.
Jeffrey E. Booth, M.D.
Brigham and Women's
   Hospital
John J. Calabro, M.D.
Jacques R. Caldwell, M.D.
Children's Hospital Medical
   Center
Children's Memorial Hospital
Ling Sun Chu, M.D.
Mack L. Clayton, M.D.
Cleveland Metropolitan
   General Hospital
Commonweal Clinic
J. Robin De Andrade, M.D.
Russell A. Del Toro, M.D.
Duke University Medical
   Center
Einstein-Moss Arthritis Center
Ephraim P. Engleman, M.D.
Albert B. Ferguson, Jr., M.D.
James F. Fries, M.D.
Germantown Hospital
Nortin M. Hadler, M.D.
Harborview Medical Center
Edward D. Harris, Jr., M.D.
Joseph Lee Hollander, M.D.
Roger Hollister, M.D.
Hospital for Joint Diseases
Hospital for Special Surgery
Gene G. Hunder, M.D.
Allan E. Inglis, M.D.
Jerry C. Jacobs, M.D.

Stephen R. Kaplan, M.D.
Valery Lanyi, M.D.
Latter Day Saints Hospital
Maimonides Medical Center
Alphonse T. Masi, M.D.
Mayo Clinic
Medical Center Sunny Isles
Medical University of South
   Carolina
Mensana Clinic
Mercy Pain Center
Montefiore Hospital Medical
   Center
Mt. Sinai Hospital
National Institutes of Health
Charles S. Neer, II, M.D.
David Neustadt, M.D.
New York University Medical
   Center
North Carolina Baptist
   Hospital and Bowman Gray
   School of Medicine
Northwestern University
   Faculty Foundation
Pain Control and Health
   Support Services
Robert H. Persellin, M.D.
James B. Peter, M.D.
Emmanuel Rudd, M.D.
St. Mary's Hospital
Peter Schur, M.D.
Robert Siffert, M.D.
Spain Rehabilitation Center
Stanford Immunology Clinic
State University Hospital,
   Downstate Medical Center
   (N.Y.)
Mary Betty Stevens, M.D.
Robert L. Swezey, M.D.
Texas Children's Hospital
Charles Tourtelotte, M.D.
University of Alabama,
   Birmingham Medical Center

University of California, Los
Angeles, School of Medicine
University of Cincinnati
Medical Center
University of Connecticut
Health Center
University of Iowa Hospital
and Clinics
University of Michigan
University of Minnesota
University of Nebraska
Hospital and Clinic
University of North Carolina
School of Medicine
University of Virginia Medical
Center
University of Washington
Medical School
Veteran's Administration
Hospital
West Virginia University
Medical Center
Robert F. Willkens, M.D.
Colin H. Wilson, Jr., M.D.
Morris Ziff, M.D.
Nathan Zvaifler, M.D.

INNOVATIVE

Robert G. Addison, M.D.
Roy D. Altman, M.D.
Arthritis and Back Pain
Center, Inc.
Arthritis and Health Resource
Center
Robert Bingham, M.D.
Sheldon Blau, M.D.
E. Richard Blonsky, M.D.
Rodney Bluestone, M.D.
Jacques R. Caldwell, M.D.
Central Mesabi Medical Center
Children's Hospital Medical
Center
Ling Sun Chu, M.D.
Mack L. Clayton, M.D.
Commonweal Clinic
Daniel Freeman Memorial
Hospital
Charles W. Denko, M.D.
Desert Arthritis Medical Clinic
Duke University Medical
Center
Einstein-Moss Arthritis Center
Emory University Pain Control
Center

Albert B. Ferguson, Jr., M.D.
James F. Fries, M.D.
Joseph Lee Hollander, M.D.
Hospital for Joint Diseases
Allan E. Inglis, M.D.
J. Hugh Kalkus, M.D.
Stephen R. Kaplan, M.D.
Lakeview Medical Clinic, S.C.
Maimonides Medical Center
Mayo Clinic
Medical Center Sunny Isles
Mensana Clinic
Mercy Hospital Medical Center
Mt. Sinai Hospital
Charles S. Neer, II, M.D.
David Neustadt, M.D.
North Carolina Baptist
Hospital and Bowman Gray
School of Medicine
Northwestern University
Faculty Foundation
Yukihiko Nosé, M.D.
Ohio Pain and Stress
Treatment Center
Pain Control and Health
Support Services
Chitranjan S. Ranawat, M.D.
Rehabilitation Institute of
Chicago
St. Joseph Clinic
James W. Smith, M.D.
Stanford University Hospital
Alfred D. Steinberg, M.D.
Robert L. Swezey, M.D.
Texas Children's Hospital
University of California, Los
Angeles, School of Medicine
University of Cincinnati
Medical Center
University of Connecticut
Health Center
University of Iowa Hospitals
and Clinics
University of Michigan
University of Nebraska
Hospital and Clinic
University of North Carolina
School of Medicine
University of Washington
Medical School
West Virginia University
Medical Center
Robert F. Willkens, M.D.

ALTERNATIVE

Acupuncture Pain Control and
  Rehabilitation Center
Robert G. Addison, M.D.
Arthritis and Health Resource
  Center
Robert C. Atkins, M.D.
Sheldon Blau, M.D.
E. Richard Blonsky, M.D.
Chenango Memorial Hospital
Children's Hospital Medical
  Center
Ling Sun Chu, M.D.
Commonweal Clinic
Coney Island Acupuncture
  Clinic
Charles W. Denko, M.D.
Desert Arthritis Medical
  Center

Lawrence D. Dickey, M.D.
Collin Dong, M.D.
Emory University Pain Control
  Center
Empire Medical Clinic
Lakeview Medical Clinic, S.C.
Maimonides Medical Center
Medical Center Sunny Isles
David Neustadt, M.D.
Pain Control and Health
  Support Services
Portland Naturopathic Clinic
St. Mary's Hospital
University of California, Los
  Angeles, School of Medicine
University of Virginia Medical
  Center
University of Washington
  Medical School
Robert F. Willkens, M.D.

ACUPUNCTURE PAIN CONTROL AND
   REHABILITATION CENTER
7227 S.W. Terwilliger
Portland, Ore. 97219
(503) 245-3156
Director: Marcelle Chiasson, M.D.

This clinic offers an alternative approach to the treatment of arthritis, according to its director. The program "consists of the use of acupuncture for pain control and to increase the body's immune system as demonstrated by Chinese researchers. . . . Physical therapy is used for muscular relaxation and counseling in a more healthy life style, including nutrition, balanced activities, and rest and proper thinking."

Treatment at this clinic is not covered by most medical insurance plans. Length of treatment varies with the individual's needs, and is on an out-patient basis only. Special financial arrangements can be made.

DR. ROBERT G. ADDISON
Center for Pain Studies
345 East Superior
Chicago, Ill. 60611
(312) 649-2845
Specialty: Orthopedics
Affiliations: Rehabilitation Institute of Chicago
       Northwestern University Medical School

Dr. Addison classifies his treatment approach as innovative and alternative. He treats the rehabilitative reduction of pain and increased mobility aspects of arthritis, especially of the spine.

If in-patient treatment is necessary, the average length of treatment is four weeks; out-patient treatment usually averages six weeks. His treatment is acceptable to most medical insurance plans, and special financial arrangements can be made by the Rehabilitation Institute.

ALFRED I. DU PONT INSTITUTE
P.O. Box 269
Wilmington, Del. 19899
(302) 651-4000
Head of Clinic: Rajeswary Padmalingam, M.D.
Affiliations: Thomas Jefferson University Medical School
              (Philadelphia)
         University of North Carolina Medical School

Dr. Padmalingam classifies the treatment approach as traditional. The program here concerns treatment of chronic juvenile arthritis, and follows a conservative course of drug therapies (salicylates, with nonsteroidal anti-inflammatories if needed), joint conservation, spondyloarthropathic treatments (with drugs and physical therapy), ophthalmological consultation, and orthopedic surgery when necessary. A team approach is used, integrating all the specialties of individual staff members into a comprehensive program.

Patients are seen on either an in- or an out-patient basis depending on the treatment course they undergo. The Institute handles up to 150 patients at any given time. Most medical insurance plans cover treatment at the institute, and special financial arrangements are possible.

DR. ROY D. ALTMAN
University of Miami School of Medicine
P.O. Box 016960 (VA111)
Miami, Fla. 33101
(305) 547-5735
Specialty: Rheumatology
Affiliations: University of Miami
              Miami Veterans' Administration Medical Center

Dr. Altman classifies his treatment approach as traditional and innovative. Most medical insurance plans cover his treatment program. No special financial arrangements are available.

DR. HARLAN AMSTUTZ
Division of Orthopedic Surgery
University of California, Los Angeles, Medical Center
Los Angeles, Calif. 90024

Dr. Amstutz is involved in research, as a grantee from NIADDK (p. 126).

ARTHRITIS AND BACK PAIN CENTER, INC.
2200 Santa Monica Boulevard
Santa Monica, Calif. 90404
(213) 829-7926
Medical Director: Dr. Robert L. Swezey

Dr. Swezey classifies the Arthritis and Back Pain Center as both traditional and innovative. Traditional diagnosis and drug therapies are used to control arthritis. What he considers innovative is the comprehensive patient education program and the integrated rehabilitation therapies, available to the patient in a setting outside a hospital. Rehabilitation includes physical and occupational therapies, and counseling services.

The treatment program is covered under most medical insurance plans, but no special financial arrangements are available.

ARTHRITIS AND HEALTH RESOURCE CENTER
486 Washington Street
Wellesley, Mass. 02181
(617) 431-7080
Director: Jeanne Lynn Melvin, MSEd, OTR

The center offers a comprehensive therapy program for people with arthritis and pain disorders. Education about the disease, rehabilitation, stress management, nutritional counseling, physical and occupational therapy, hand therapy, and exercise/conditioning classes are among the components of the program. The director calls it a "wellness center that provides a wide range of programs which enable people to apply an holistic health perspective to their lives." The services are available to adults, adolescents, parents and family of patients, and health professionals.

Fees are on a treatment basis, ranging from $10/hour for group treatment sessions to $50/hour for some of the individual therapies. Some of the programs are covered by insurance plans; check with your insurance carrier. As of this writing, Medicare does not cover treatment at the center.

DR. ROBERT C. ATKINS
400 East 56th Street
New York, N.Y. 10022
(212) 758-2110

Dr. Atkins' practice has evolved into a nutritionally oriented treatment program. Although he does not specialize in rheumatology, Dr. Atkins treats arthritis on an individual basis. The focus is on the patient's nutritional needs. These are determined by the appropriate laboratory tests.

DR. PETER BARLAND
Montefiore Medical Center
111 East 210th Street
Bronx, N.Y. 10467
(212) 920-5455
Specialties: Internal Medicine, Rheumatology
Affiliations: Montefiore Medical Center
            Albert Einstein College of Medicine

Dr. Barland classifies his treatment approach as traditional. His treatment program begins with a thorough examination including a complete history, physical exam, laboratory testing, and X-rays. Patient education is stressed.

In patients with forms of arthritis resistant to conservative treatment, short courses of intensive plasmapheresis (p. 40) are sometimes used.

Treatment can take anywhere from months to years, depending on the severity of the illness, although Dr. Barland does not hospitalize patients as a part of his treatment program. Most medical insurance plans will cover his treatment, but no special financial arrangements are available.

DR. JOHN BAUM
Monroe Community Hospital
435 East Henrietta Road
Rochester, N.Y. 14603
(716) 473-4080, ext. 367
Specialty: Rheumatology
Affiliations: University of Rochester School of Medicine
Strong Memorial Hospital
Monroe Community Hospital

Dr. Baum takes a traditional approach in treating the rheumatic diseases. Length of treatment varies. Hospitalization for a period of up to three weeks is necessary on occasion. Most medical insurance plans cover the treatment, and special financial arrangements are possible.

DR. ROBERT BINGHAM
Suite 301
1000 South Anaheim Boulevard
Anaheim, Calif. 92805
(714) 776-3222
Specialty: Orthopedic Surgery
Affiliation: Desert Arthritis Medical Clinic

Dr. Bingham's approach to the treatment of arthritis involves using natural methods and a nutritional program. (See also *Desert Arthritis Medical Clinic*, p. 91.)

DR. SHELDON BLAU
566 Broadway, N-11
Massapequa, N.Y. 11758
(516) 541-6262
Specialty: Rheumatology
Affiliations: Clinical Professor of Medicine, State University
of New York, Downstate Medical Center
Chief of Rheumatology, Nassau County Medical
Center
Chief of Arthritis Clinic, Nassau Hospital

Dr. Blau classifies his treatment approach as traditional, innovative, and alternative. Pragmatism is stressed.

Treatment with Dr. Blau may range from a few hours to an ongoing, long-term program, depending on the form of rheumatic disease and its severity. Hospitalization occurs rarely. Most medical insurance plans cover his treatment, and special financial arrangements are possible

DR. E. RICHARD BLONSKY
Center for Pain Studies
345 East Superior
Chicago, Ill. 60611
(312) 649-2845
Specialty: Neurology
Affiliations: Rehabilitation Institute of Chicago
Northwestern University Medical School.

Dr. Blonsky, who is in practice with Dr. Robert Addison (p. 81), classifies his treatment approach as innovative and alternative. He specializes in treating the spine.

Out-patient treatment lasts an average of six weeks, whereas if hospitalization is required, the period involved is usually four weeks. Most medical insurance plans cover treatment at the Center for Pain Studies. Special financial arrangements are available.

DR. RODNEY BLUESTONE
8631 West Third Street
Los Angeles, Calif. 90048
(213) 657-2222
Specialty: Rheumatology
Affiliation: Clinical Professor of Medicine, University of
California, Los Angeles

Classifying his treatment approach as innovative, Dr. Bluestone incorporates new methods and drugs in his treatment of arthritis.

Average length of treatment with Dr. Bluestone is six months, with hospitalization occasionally required. The length of hospitalization in those cases most often is one to two weeks. His treatments are covered by most medical insurance plans, but no special financial arrangements are available.

DR. JEFFREY E. BOOTH
3905 Harrison Boulevard, #508
Ogden, Utah 84403
(801) 399-4431
Specialty: Rheumatology
Affiliations: Ogden Arthritis Associates
Clinical faculty of University of Utah Medical
School
McKay Dee Hospital Rehabilitation Center

Dr. Booth's treatment approach, as he classifies it, is "traditional, and evolving with new research discoveries." He will hospitalize patients, when needed, for an average stay of 10 to 14 days. Most of these hospitalizations are on the rehabilitation unit, when patients need concentrated medical attention, physical therapy, occupational therapy, psychological guidance, and/or the help of a social worker in connection with their illness. Medical insurance plans cover Dr. Booth's treatment.

BRIGHAM AND WOMEN'S HOSPITAL
The Ambulatory Center
Robert B. Brigham Division
75 Francis Street
Boston, Mass. 02115
(617) 732-5320
Director: K. Frank Austen, M.D.

This "traditional" treatment center has two special clinics, one for lupus patients, the other for juvenile arthritis patients. The accepted, conservative drug therapies are practiced. The center treats both in- and out-patients; 19,000 patients are treated per year.

Treatment at the center is covered by most medical insurance plans, and special financial arrangements are possible.

DR. JOHN J. CALABRO
Saint Vincent Hospital
25 Winthrop Street
Worcester, Mass. 01604
(617) 798-6125/6130
Specialty: Rheumatology
Affiliations: Director of Rheumatology, Saint Vincent
               Hospital
               Professor of Medicine and Pediatrics, University
               of Massachusetts Medical School (Worcester)

Dr. Calabro classifies his treatment approach as traditional. He stresses the need for patient education in order to foster cooperation. He says that "Patient education is clearly the cornerstone of all successful chronic disease management."

The large majority of his patients are seen on an out-patient basis; only one or two percent are hospitalized. Average treatment length runs from two to four years. Special financial arrangements are possible, and most medical insurance plans cover treatment by Dr. Calabro.

DR. JACQUES R. CALDWELL
7106 N.W. 11th Place,
Gainesville, Fla. 32605
(904) 377-4522
Specialities: Internal Medicine, Rheumatology, Allergy
Affiliation: Clinical Associate Professor of Medicine,
              Department of Medicine, University of Florida
              School of Medicine

Dr. Caldwell describes his treatment approach as traditional and innovative. He has written and lectured extensively on arthritis, dealing with the topics of drug therapies, allergic response and its involvement in acute inflammation, medical management of rheumatoid arthritis, and immune deficiencies, among others.

CENTRAL MESABI MEDICAL CENTER
Acupuncture and Pain Clinic
750 East 34th Street
Hibbing, Minn. 55746
(218) 262-4881
Director: William C. Lee, M.D.

This clinic offers an innovative treatment approach, according to Dr. Lee. The treatment method is either auriculotherapy (ear acupuncture) or traditional body acupuncture. Treatment averages three weeks, on an out-patient basis. Most medical insurance plans do not cover treatment at this clinic, but special financial arrangements are possible.

CHENANGO MEMORIAL HOSPITAL
Acupuncture Clinic
Experimental Medicine and Research Clinic
R.D. #3, Box 480
Norwich, N.Y. 13815
(607) 334-9994
Director: Primitivo T. Cruz, M.D. (licensed by the state of
          New York for acupuncture on a research basis)

Patients to this clinic are usually referred by their attending physicians. As Dr. Cruz explains, "These patients, as a rule, have been treated with all modalities available to Western medicine . . . but still suffer from persistent pain. A history and physical exam are done on the first visit. Traditional meridian points are located corresponding to the regional disease being treated, and needles are put in place and left for 20 minutes. There is an attending nurse at all times with the patient."

For those patients who are unable to tolerate the needles, a transcutaneous electro-neurostimulator, which gives a mild electrical impulse that stimulates the nerves, is used. Dr. Cruz has treated patients with rheumatoid arthritis and degenerative osteoarthritis, involving various joints.

Treatment is on an out-patient basis only, with three to four treatments per week. Medical insurance plans do not cover this treatment program, nor are special financial arrangements available.

CHILDREN'S HOSPITAL MEDICAL CENTER
Special Treatment Center for Juvenile Arthritis
Convalescent and Services Pavilion, Room 1-29
Elland and Bethesda Avenues
Cincinnati, Ohio 45229
(513) 559-4676
Affiliations: Children's Hospital Medical Center,
              Division of Pediatric Rheumatology
              University of Cincinnati Medical School,
              Division of Immunology

This treatment center is both traditional and alternative in its approach to the treatment of arthritis. It employs "a multidisciplinary team approach, interacting with the patient and family in a coordinated and comprehensive way. The rheumatic diseases of childhood are diagnosed according to established criteria. Patients are seen as required for specific therapeutic reasons and at intervals of six to 12 months for clinical reassessment and outcome evaluation. These periodic reviews include complete physical examinations, appropriate laboratory studies, X rays, reinforcement and modification of physical therapy instructions and techniques, assessments of activities of daily living, and psychosocial and career development, and family and financial counseling as indicated." Patients are followed from the onset of their disease into adult life.

Hospitalization is infrequent. Treatment at the center is covered by most medical insurance plans, and special financial arrangements are possible.

CHILDREN'S MEMORIAL HOSPITAL
Arthritis Pediatric Center
2300 Children's Plaza
Chicago, Ill. 60614
(312) 880-4360
Head of Division: Lauren M. Pachman, M.D.
Affiliation: Northwestern Medical Center

The Children's Memorial Hospital Immunology/Rheumatology Clinic has nearly 2,000 pediatric visits per year; about 250 of these are new patients. Patients may be referred by their doctors or by the Arthritis Foundation, or may decide to come without referral. The Arthritis Pediatric Center uses a team approach; the staff includes two rheumatologists, an orthopedic surgeon, ophthalmologist, physical therapist, occupational therapist, nurse clinician, and social worker (Spanish/English speaking). The treatment addresses four areas: medical, psychosocial, educational, and research.

The average length of treatment depends on the severity of a given patient's condition, and may last for years. Patients are seen on an in- or an out-patient basis, depending on their condition. Most medical insurance plans cover treatment at the clinic, and special financial arrangements are possible.

DR. LING SUN CHU
107 East 73rd Street
New York, N.Y. 10021
(212) 472-3000
Specialties: Internal Medicine and Acupuncture

Dr. Chu's treatment program entails the use of drug therapy, physical therapy, and acupuncture. He may refer a patient for surgery, as well.

Most medical insurance plans cover Dr. Chu's treatment program, but no special financial arrangements are available.

DR. MACK L. CLAYTON
2005 Franklin, #550
Denver, Colo. 80205
(303) 839-5383
Specialties: Orthopedics, Arthritis reconstructive surgery
Affiliations: Denver Orthopedic Clinic
          St. Joseph and Rose Medical Center Hospitals
          Clinical Professor of Surgery, Associate Clinical
          Professor of Orthopedic Surgery, University
          of Colorado

Dr. Clayton classifies his treatment approach as traditional and innovative, stating that he and his associates "have developed surgery fitted into a 'team approach,' in cooperation with rheumatology and allied health specialists as necessary." His specialty is hand surgery, an area in which there are many new advances.

Hospitalization is usually one to two weeks in duration, with follow-up visits after that. Most medical insurance plans cover Dr. Clayton's treatment, and special financial arrangements are possible.

CLEVELAND METROPOLITAN GENERAL HOSPITAL
Arthritis Clinic
3395 Scranton Road
Cleveland, Ohio 44109
(216) 398-6000
Affiliation: Case Western Reserve University

Traditional treatment is practiced at this clinic. Along with the pharmacological therapies (pp. 26–42), occupational therapy, physical therapy, and psychological counseling are employed as part of the overall treatment program.

Treatment is covered by most medical insurance plans, and special financial arrangements can be made. Patients are seen on an in- or an out-patient basis, depending upon their condition.

COMMONWEAL CLINIC
451 Mesa Road
P.O. Box 316
Bolinas, Calif. 94924
(415) 868-1501
Director: Lester Adler, M.D.

Dr. Adler classifies this clinic as taking both a traditional and an alternative approach to the treatment of arthritis. Nutritional and vitamin therapy are important parts of the clinic's program. Treatment usually consists of three or four visits, unless there are psychological problems involved, or complications requiring more time. All patients are seen as out-patients only.

Most medical insurance plans cover the treatment at Commonweal Clinic, and special financial arrangements are possible.

CONEY ISLAND ACUPUNCTURE CLINIC
2802 Mermaid Avenue
Brooklyn, N.Y. 11224
(212) 372-4569
Director: Leo Wollman, M.D.

This clinic is alternative in its approach. The only treatment modality is acupuncture. Treatment, which is on an out-patient basis only, averages six weeks in duration. Most medical insurance plans do not cover this therapy, and special financial arrangements are not available.

DANIEL FREEMAN MEMORIAL HOSPITAL
Center for Diagnostic and Rehabilitative Medicine
Rheumatic Disease Rehabilitation Program
333 North Prairie Avenue
Inglewood, Calif. 90301
(213) 674-7050, ext. 3238
Director: James B. Peter, M.D.
Affiliation: University of California, Los Angeles, School of
          Medicine

Dr. Peter classifies this program as innovative. Treatment is "of the patient as a whole person, with emphasis on improvement of function and preventive approaches." Education is an important part of the treatment.

The program takes three weeks, beginning with time as an in-patient; after the testing and evaluation is complete, the patient continues as an out-patient. Most medical insurance plans cover treatment in this program, and special financial arrangements are possible.

DR. J. ROBIN DE ANDRADE
Emory University Clinic
1365 Clifton Road, N.E.
Atlanta, Ga. 30322
(404) 321-0111
Specialty: Orthopedics
Affiliation: Emory University Medical School

Dr. De Andrade classifies his treatment as traditional, involving "surgical management of arthritis." Hospitalization averages 14 days, although the total length of treatment is indefinite, depending on the severity of the individual patient's condition.

Most medical insurance plans cover Dr. De Andrade's treatment program, and special financial arrangements can be made.

DR. RUSSELL A. DEL TORO
Ashford Medical Center, 809
Santurce, Puerto Rico 00907
(809) 723-6225
Specialties: Rheumatology, Internal Medicine
Affiliation: University of Puerto Rico School of Medicine

Dr. Del Toro's approach to the treatment of arthritis is primarily traditional. Hospitalization is not usually required in his treatment plan. The average length of treatment varies according to the patient's condition.

Dr. Del Toro's treatments are covered by most medical insurance plans; he specifies that he accepts direct payment from the patient, who then is reimbursed by the insurance company. Special financial arrangements are possible.

DR. CHARLES W. DENKO
George Scott Research Labs
Fairview General Hospital
18101 Lorain Avenue
Cleveland, Ohio 44111
(216) 476-7188
Specialty: Rheumatology
Affiliations: Fairview General Hospital
            Case Western Reserve University

Dr. Denko is quite specific in classifying his approach to the treatment of arthritis. For osteoarthritis, he says he has an "innovative" approach, while for rheumatoid arthritis he used the "alternative" classification.

Treatment length differs according to the condition being treated: osteoarthritis averages one to two years, whereas an acute case of rheumatoid arthritis takes one to two weeks to treat. Chronic rheumatoid arthritis is treated indefinitely, according to the patient's needs. Hospitalization is not considered necessary for osteoarthritis, but it may be for rheumatoid arthritis.

Most medical insurance plans cover Dr. Denko's treatment programs, and special financial arrangements are possible.

DESERT ARTHRITIS MEDICAL CLINIC
13-630 Mountain View Road
Desert Hot Springs, Calif. 92240
(619) 329-6422
Director: Robert Bingham, M.D.
Affiliation: Esperanza Intercommunity Hospital (Yorba
            Linda, Calif.)

Dr. Bingham classifies the clinic's treatment approach as innovative and alternative. He summarizes the philosophy of the clinic: "We have discovered that 60 percent of all arthritis patients can be improved by correcting dietary deficiencies, eliminating allergic foods, and avoiding certain toxic substances in the diets." This program has been in effect for more than 17 years; in addition to the methods outlined above, the Desert Arthritis Medical Clinic uses natural methods of physical therapy. Full blood work-ups are conducted to determine the state of the body and blood chemistries, and other laboratory and medical tests are run. The average length of treatment is two to three weeks, on an out-patient basis only.

Another facet of the program is the administration of yucca herbal extract, a substance Dr. Bingham and his staff have found to be of great value in treating arthritis. They also use some procedures and drug therapies that, they claim, are as effective as the conventional medications, without the side effects. These include: a special "arthritis vaccine" that improves the patient's natural immunity and resistance against arthritis; antiprotozoal medications (pioneered in England by Dr. Roger Wyburn-Mason) that remove the cause of some forms of rheumatoid arthritis; electro-acupuncture; and joint aspiration and injections.

There is also a surgical treatment program available through the clinic.

A large portion of the costs at the clinic is covered by most insurance plans or Medicare. Each patient should check with his/ her insurance carrier.

DR. LAWRENCE D. DICKEY
109 West Olive Street
Ft. Collins, Colo. 80524
(303) 482-6001
Specialty: Clinical Ecology

Dr. Dickey is one of the early clinical ecologists. He treats his patients according to the principles of that specialty (pp. 49–51).

DR. COLLIN DONG
950 Stockton
San Francisco, Calif. 94108
(415) 982-2872
Specialty: Internal Medicine

Dr. Dong, trained as an orthodox physician, has evolved a practice based on diet, rather than on medications and/or surgery, to treat the symptoms and effects of rheumatic disease (pp. 52–53). His diet eliminates many foods that, he claims, irritate the system.

Dr. Dong's diet is explained in great detail (with recipes included) in two books, *The Arthritic's Cookbook* and *New Hope for the Arthritic.* Both are sold in bookstores and are available in libraries.

DUKE UNIVERSITY MEDICAL CENTER
Rheumatology Clinic
P.O. Box 3892
Durham, N.C. 27710
(919) 684-6205
Director: Ralph Snyderman, M.D.
Affiliation: Duke University School of Medicine

The treatment approach here is both traditional and innovative. Conventional treatments are followed for the control of the disease, and more innovative methods are employed in treating chronic pain. Some of these methods include biofeedback and transcutaneous electro-neurostimulators, which use mild electric shock to stimulate the nerves.

Treatment is on both an in- and an out-patient basis. Most medical insurance plans cover treatment at the clinic, and special financial arrangements are possible.

EINSTEIN-MOSS ARTHRITIS CENTER
Korman Building, #103
York and Tabor Roads
Philadelphia, Pa. 19141
(215) 456-7380
Head of Center: Mary E. Moore, M.D., Ph.D.
Affiliation: Temple University

Dr. Moore classifies the Einstein-Moss Arthritis Center as both traditional and innovative. She says the center "makes available on one campus a unique combination of out-patient office care; acute in-patient treatment . . . and specialized hospitalization for rehabilitation in a small, fully equipped rehabilitation hospital. . . .[It] also provides an unusually complete multidisciplinary approach to the care of the arthritic."

The staff at the center includes rheumatologists, orthopedic surgeons, and therapy specialists, as well as physiatrists (specialists in rehabilitative medicine), psychologists, social workers, and clinical nurse specialists.

Treatment takes two to three weeks on the average. Treatment is covered by most medical insurance plans, and special financial arrangements can be made.

EMORY UNIVERSITY PAIN CONTROL CENTER
Center of Rehabilitation Medicine
1441 Clifton Road, N.E.
Atlanta, Ga. 30322
(404) 329-5492
Director: Steven F. Brena, M.D.
Affiliation: Emory University

Dr. Brena classifies the treatment approach here as innovative and alternative. His description states that the approach is "physio-psychological rehabilitation to restore—or to improve—patients' skills to cope with the chronic arthritic conditions. Methodology is mostly based on behavior modification."

The program is a two-week in-patient plan, although for a selected few it can be on an out-patient basis. Most medical insurance plans cover the treatment program here, and special financial arrangements are possible.

EMPIRE MEDICAL CLINIC
E17 Empire
Spokane, Wash. 99207
(509) 328-3430
Director: Hi Young Lee, M.D.

This clinic combines acupuncture with traditional treatments. Patients are seen on an out-patient basis only, and treatment length varies according to the patient's needs.

Most medical insurance plans do not cover the acupuncture treatment, although the traditional aspects of the program may be covered. Check with your insurance carrier.

DR. EPHRAIM P. ENGLEMAN
University of California Medical Center
San Francisco, Calif. 94143
(415) 666-1141
Specialty: Rheumatology
Affiliation: University of California, San Francisco

Dr. Engleman classifies his treatment approach as traditional, using "conservative anti-inflammatory and pain-reducing drugs, appropriate exercise and joint protection, and orthopedic surgery when indicated." Accordingly, the average length of treatment may be years. There usually is no hospitalization involved. Treatment is covered by most medical insurance plans, but no special financial arrangements are available.

DR. ALBERT B. FERGUSON, JR.
3601 Fifth Avenue
Pittsburgh, Pa 15213
(412) 681-3604
Specialty: Orthopedic surgery
Affiliation: University of Pittsburgh Medical Center

Dr. Ferguson calls his treatment approach traditional and innovative. He performs artifical joint surgery. Hospitalization for his treatment usually lasts seven days. Most medical insurance plans cover Dr. Ferguson's treatment, but no special financial arrangements are available.

DR. JAMES F. FRIES
Division of Immunology
Stanford University Hospital
Stanford University
Stanford, Calif. 94305
(415) 497-6003
Specialty: Rheumatology
Affiliations: Stanford University
              Clinical Director, Division of Immunology,
              Stanford University Hospital

Dr. Fries classifies his treatment approach as traditional and innovative. He believes that patient education is an important part of the process of helping the patient. Treatment varies in length, depending upon the particular problem and its complexity.
Dr. Fries does not hospitalize patients as part of the treatment. All medical insurance plans cover his work; only rarely are special financial arrangements possible.

GERMANTOWN HOSPITAL
Rheumatology Associates
2 Penn Boulevard
Philadelphia, Pa. 19144
(215) 844-1118
Affiliation: Temple University

The treatment approach here is traditional. Patients are seen on both an in-and an out-patient basis; the program is tailored to the individual's needs. Most medical insurance plans cover this treatment regimen, and special financial arrangements are possible.

DR. NORTIN M. HADLER
Department of Medicine
University of North Carolina School of Medicine
Chapel Hill, N.C. 27514
(919) 966-4191
Specialties: Rheumatology, Internal Medicine, Allergy and
  Clinical Immunology
Affiliations: North Carolina Memorial Hospital
  University of North Carolina School of
  Medicine

Dr. Hadler considers his approach to the treatment of arthritis to be traditional. He says that treatment "depends on the patient and his/her illness," referring to both length and actual course of treatment. Hospitalization may or may not be required.

Dr. Hadler's treatment program is covered by most medical insurance plans. Special financial arrangements can be made, if necessary.

HARBORVIEW MEDICAL CENTER
Harborview Arthritis Clinic
325 Ninth Avenue
Seattle, Wash. 98104
(206) 223-3156
Director: Robert F. Willkens, M.D.

This clinic, sponsored in part by the National Institutes of Health (p. 103) and by the Arthritis Foundation (p. 127), is traditional in its approach, but innovative treatment methods and therapeutic drugs are also part of its program. Diagnostic services are an important part of the clinic's function as well.

DR. JOSEPH LEE HOLLANDER
3400 Spruce Street
Philadelphia, Pa 19104
(215) 662-2454
Specialties: Internal Medicine; Rheumatology
Affiliation: Emeritus Professor of Medicine, University of
  Pennsylvania School of Medicine

Dr. Hollander classifies his treatment approach as both traditional and innovative. Acknowledging his understanding that most forms of arthritis are both chronic and incurable, he states his belief that "function can be preserved" through the use of various medications and physical techniques.

Treatment length depends on the type of arthritis, and hospitalization is sometimes a part of his treatment method. Dr. Hollander's treatments are covered by most medical insurance plans, and special financial arrangements are possible.

DR. ROGER HOLLISTER
National Jewish Hospital/National Asthma Center
3800 East Colfax Avenue
Denver, Colo. 80206
(303) 398-1378
Specialty: Rheumatology
Affiliation: University of Colorado School of Medicine

Dr. Hollister classifies his treatment approach as traditional. He prefers to use aspirin and the nonsteroidal anti-inflammatories (p. 27) to combat the inflammation of arthritis, but if necessary, he will prescribe gold or penicillamine for those patients who are unresponsive to the more conservative therapy.

His treatment program includes physical and/or occupational therapy, and school counseling on an out-patient basis for those who need it. His pediatric patients are admitted to the pediatric rehabilitation service at the hospital if their condition warrants. This service may include surgery. Stress is placed on handling "problems with age-appropriate techniques."

Other than this rehabilitative aspect, Dr. Hollister's treatment does not involve hospitalization. Most medical insurance plans cover his treatment program, and special financial arrangements can be made.

HOSPITAL FOR JOINT DISEASES
Orthopaedic-Arthritis Pain Center
Orthopaedic Institute
301 East 17th Street
New York, N.Y. 10003
(212) 598-6606
Director: Isaac Pinter, Ph.D.
Affiliation: Mt. Sinai School of Medicine

Dr. Pinter describes the center's program as innovative. The primary purpose and focus is "to provide a comprehensive approach to the care of. . .rheumatological patients suffering from chronic disabling musculoskeletal pain." To that effect, the pain center's approach is to eliminate harmful drugs, to treat the psychological and physiological symptoms that often accompany intractable pain, and to modify physical and mental behavior to allow the patients to assume a useful and gratifying role in society, as well as to relieve pain. The center uses automated psychological testing, which allows the doctors to formulate a more precise diagnosis and treatment plan.

Initial referral is for evaluation only. Once accepted into the program, the patient spends the first three weeks as an in-patient and the next 23 weeks as an out-patient. The program is entirely voluntary and may be terminated at any point in the six month period at the patient's request.

Most insurance plans cover treatment at the Center, and special financial arrangements are possible.

HOSPITAL FOR SPECIAL SURGERY
535 East 71st Street
New York, N.Y. 10021
(212) 606-1000
Physician-in-Chief: Charles Christian, M.D.
Affiliation: Cornell Medical Center

The hospital administrator classifies the treatment approach as traditional. It is a teaching facility for orthopedic and rheumatological conditions. Patients are seen on an in- or an out-patient basis, depending on their condition.

There is a Pain Service, which accepts patients on referral from other physicians. Treatment here, too, is on both an in- and an out-patient basis. Among the procedures used are biofeedback, drug therapies, nutritional counseling and therapy, relaxation techniques, transcutaneous electric nerve stimulation (p. 87), and various forms of psychological counseling.

Length of treatment at the hospital varies according to the disease. Most medical insurance plans cover treatment at the hospital, and special financial arrangements are possible, depending on circumstances.

DR. GENE G. HUNDER
200 First Street, S.W.
Rochester, Minn. 55905
(507) 284-3511
Specialties: Internal Medicine, Rheumatology
Affiliations: Mayo Clinic
Professor of Medicine, Mayo Medical School

Dr. Hunder says, "I use the traditional forms of treatment for various kinds of arthritic disease. Depending on the disease and its complexity, length of treatment varies. If hospitalization is warranted, the patient's stay can be from one to four weeks in duration; this, too, is determined by the patient's condition."

Dr. Hunder's treatment program is covered by most medical insurance plans, and special financial arrangements are possible.

DR. ALLAN E. INGLIS
Hospital for Special Surgery
535 East 70th Street
New York, N.Y. 10021
(212) 606-1335
Specialty: Orthopedic Surgery: Surgery of Arthritis
Affiliations: Hospital for Special Surgery
Cornell University Medical College

Dr. Inglis describes his treatment as both innovative and traditional. He seeks to correct "hip, knee, foot, hand, wrist, elbow, shoulder, and cervical spine deformities" using surgery. Hospitalization for any of these treatments averages 14 days, and follow-up appointments are necessary. Medical insurance plans usually cover this kind of surgery. Special financial arrangements may be made.

DR. JERRY C. JACOBS
4621 Waldo Avenue
Riverdale, N.Y. 10471
(212) 548-5431
Specialty: Pediatric Rheumatology
Affiliations: Professor of Clinical Pediatrics, Columbia
              University College of Physicians and
              Surgeons
              Director, Section of Pediatric Rheumatology,
              Columbia-Presbyterian Medical Center

Dr. Jacobs classifies his treatment approach as traditional, with his goal in all cases being "normal function for arthritic children." Treatment varies in length according to the patient's needs, but hospitalization is not part of Dr. Jacob's program. Most medical insurance plans cover his treatment, but no special financial arrangements are possible.

In addition to his office in Riverdale, Dr. Jacobs has an office at Columbia-Presbyterian Medical Center. The telephone number there is (212) 694-5514.

DR. J. HUGH KALKUS
Fife Medical Office
5619 Valley Avenue, East
Tacoma, Wash. 98424
(206) 922-0311
Specialties: Arthritis, Hypnotherapy, and General Practice

Dr. Kalkus classifies his treatment program as innovative. He uses various protocols, depending on the individual patient's condition. Vaccine injections (both bacterial and viral) are administered to stimulate the immune system. Hormone injections may also be used. Hypnosis is employed, when indicated, in order to relieve the tension, pain, and general stress that arthritis causes its victims.

Treatment depends on the patient's response. There is no hospitalization. Most medical insurance plans cover Dr. Kalkus' treatment program, and special financial arrangements can be made.

DR. STEPHEN R. KAPLAN
825 Chalkstone Avenue
Providence, R.I. 02908
(401) 456-2069
Specialty: Rheumatology
Affiliations: Rheumatology Center, Roger Williams General
              Hospital
              Brown University Program in Medicine

Dr. Kaplan classifies his approach to the treatment of arthritis as traditional and innovative. Treatment length varies according to the patient's condition; patients may be hospitalized. Most medical insurance plans cover Dr. Kaplan's treatment, and special financial arrangements are possible.

LAKEVIEW MEDICAL CLINIC, S.C.
2830 Dryden Drive
Madison, Wis. 53704
(608) 241-3451
Director: Christopher Gencheff, M.D.

Dr. Gencheff classifies the clinic's treatment approach as innovative and alternative. The treatment includes acupuncture and osteopathic manipulative therapy. Dr. Gencheff states: "Very often if the arthritic patient cannot tolerate medicines we employ the art of acupuncture to help control and even turn off pain. Everything is explained and a full history with physical exam is given before the treatments are given or begun on the initial visit. Very often, the treatments reduce the pain in two to four visits depending on the patient. . . ."

Treatment is handled strictly on an out-patient basis; the first visit lasts from one to one and a half hours, with subsequent treatments lasting for about 25 minutes. Not all forms of treatment are covered by medical insurance plans, but special financial arrangements can be made.

DR. VALERY LANYI
45 East 85th Street
New York, N.Y. 10028
(212) 772-1212
Specialties: Physical Medicine, Rehabilitation
Affiliations: Clinical Professor of Rehabilitation Medicine,
            New York University Medical Center
            Director of Rehabilitation, St. Clare's Hospital

In addition to practicing rehabilitation medicine, Dr. Lanyi has been doing clinical research and teaching related to rehabilitation of arthritic patients. Average length of treatment is several months, with hospitalization lasting an average of six weeks. Treatment is covered by most medical insurance plans.

LATTER DAY SAINTS HOSPITAL
Salt Lake Clinic
333 South Ninth, East
Salt Lake City, Utah 84102
(801) 535-8182
Affiliation: University of Utah College of Medicine

This clinic has a traditional approach to the treatment of arthritis. A specific diagnosis is made on the basis of a complete history, a physical exam, and appropriate laboratory tests. Medications and rehabilitative therapies are then prescribed. Surgery may be performed.

Treatment length varies with the individual. Most patients are seen and treated as out-patients. Treatment at the clinic is covered by most medical insurance plans; no special financial arrangements are available.

MAIMONIDES MEDICAL CENTER
Pain Therapy Center
4802 10th Avenue
Brooklyn, N.Y. 11219
(212) 270-7177
Director: Philip H. Sechzer, M.D.
Affiliation: State University of New York, Downstate
Medical Center

This center uses both traditional and alternative approaches in treating arthritis. Acupuncture is often part of the program and is the only therapy that is not covered by medical insurance plans. No special financial arrangements are available.

DR. ALPHONSE T. MASI
Department of Medicine
University of Illinois College of Medicine at Peoria
P.O. Box 1649
Peoria, Ill. 61656
(309) 671-3019
Specialties: Internal Medicine, Rheumatology
Affiliations: Methodist Medical Center
St. Francis Medical Center
University of Illinois College of Medicine at
Peoria

Dr. Masi classifies his treatment approach as traditional. One aspect of this approach is behavior modification, which is used in conjunction with the appropriate drugs or procedures.

Treatment length varies with each patient, depending on the individual's condition. Hospitalization is rarely required. Medical insurance plans cover Dr. Masi's treatment, and special financial arrangements are possible.

MAYO CLINIC
Pain Clinic
200 First Street, S.W.
Rochester, Minn. 55901
(507) 284-2511
Head of Pain Clinic: Josef K. Wang, M.D.
Affiliation: Mayo Medical School

Dr. Wang classifies the clinics' approach as innovative. The program begins with a thorough diagnosis. Once the diagnosis is determined, a patient may be treated with pharmacological modalities, physiotherapy, joint injections (if the condition warrants), counseling, acupuncture for relief of symptomatic pain, and/or reconstructive orthopedic surgery. It is a comprehensive program, conducted on an out-patient basis (unless surgery is indicated).

The treatment at the clinic lasts from one to two weeks. Patients are often expected to continue with medication and exercise programs at home. The clinic can handle about 20 patients a day. Most medical insurance plans cover treatment at the clinic (check about the acupuncture, however, as it may not be covered), and special financial arrangements are possible.

MEDICAL CENTER SUNNY ISLES
Department of Holistic Medicine
18600 Collins Avenue
Miami Beach, Fla. 33160
(305) 931-8484
Director: Martin Dayton, D.O.M.D.

Dr. Dayton classifies this program as traditional, innovative, and alternative in its approach. Each patient's program is determined according to the individual's condition and needs. Conventional therapies include drugs, orthopedics, osteopathic manipulative therapy, and physical therapy. Dr. Dayton also practices what he calls "holistic" modalities, which include diet evaluation, nutrition, chelation, exercise, acupuncture, allergy orthomolecular, herbal, homeopathy, biofeedback, and lifestyle evaluation and modification.

All patients are seen on an out-patient basis; treatment length varies depending on the patient's progress. Most medical insurance plans cover the treatment at the center, although some of the holistic treatment may not be included in coverage.

MEDICAL UNIVERSITY OF SOUTH CAROLINA
Arthritis Center
171 Ashley Avenue
Charleston, S.C. 29425
(803) 792-4152
Director: E.C. LeRoy, M.D.
Affiliation: Medical University of South Carolina, School of
Medicine

Dr. LeRoy calls the treatment approach here "multidisciplinary." A group of rheumatologists use a team approach to treat a wide range of rheumatic disease problems.

Length of treatment varies according to the problem being treated; some patients may be hospitalized. Treatment is covered by most medical insurance plans.

MENSANA CLINIC
1718 Greenspring Valley Road
Stevenson, Md. 21153
(301) 653-2403
Director: Nelson Hendler, M.D.

Dr. Hendler classifies this clinic as both traditional and innovative in its approach to the treatment of arthritis pain. It is a multidisciplinary treatment center for the management of pain. The clinic's staff makes every effort to make the "chronic pain sufferer more functional." Among the tools used are physical therapy, saunas, whirlpool, biofeedback, exercise, transcutaneous electric nerve stimulation (p. 87), trigger point injections, and group and/or individual psychotherapy. The emphasis on rehabilitating the patient includes the elimination of narcotic and/or hypnotic drugs.

Mensana Clinic requires physician referral for evaluation of a patient; suitability for treatment is determined by past treatment history as well as by the patient's condition. The patients in the program stay within the confines of the clinic to afford the "convenience of seeing the clinicians daily." Treatment lasts an average of three to four weeks. Clinical fees are covered by most medical insurance plans, and special financial arrangements are possible.

MERCY HOSPITAL MEDICAL CENTER
Mercy Pain Center
Sixth and University
Des Moines, Iowa 50314
(515) 247-4430
Head of Mercy Pain Center: James L. Blessman, M.D.

Dr. Blessman states that this program is "innovative" in its approach to the treatment of arthritis pain. Although traditional therapies are part of the treatment, and a rheumatologist is on staff, nutrition plays an integral role in Mercy Pain Center's program. Dietary instruction and counseling are given to each patient on an individual basis, and there are group instruction sessions as well.

Physical therapy in the form of aquatic exercises in a therapeutic pool is also used extensively. The program runs a total of three to four weeks per patient, and is on an out-patient basis. The patient load is 20 patients per session. The treatment day begins at 7:45 a.m. every week day, ending at 8:30 p.m. Monday through Thursday and at 3 p.m. on Friday. The program is acceptable to major medical plans, and special financial arrangements can be made.

MONTEFIORE HOSPITAL MEDICAL CENTER
Arthritis Clinic
111 East 210th Street
Bronx, N.Y. 10467
(212) 920-4321

The treatment program here is comprehensive and traditional. Careful diagnosis of the patient's condition is arrived at by use of appropriate laboratory testing and a thorough physical examination and history. Medication, physical and occupational therapies, and counseling are all determined on a case-by-case basis. Most medical insurance plans cover the treatment here.

MONTEFIORE HOSPITAL MEDICAL CENTER
Pain Treatment Center
111 East 210th Street
Bronx, N.Y. 10467
(212) 920-4440
Director: Edith Kepes, M.D.

Patients are referred to the Pain Treatment Center from the Arthritis Clinic if *pain* is not manageable. At the pain treatment center, patients' medications are evaluated, along with their emotional state. Treatment here may include antidepressives, biofeedback, psychotherapy, physiotherapy, transcutaneous electric nerve stimulation (p. 87), and relaxation techniques.

Treatment usually lasts from three to 12 visits, after which the patient continues his or her individualized program at home. Treatment is strictly on an out-patient basis. Most medical plans cover the program here, but no special financial arrangements are available.

MT. SINAI HOSPITAL
Arthritis Clinic
1 East 100th Street
New York, N.Y. 10029
(212) 650-6500
Director of Clinic: Selvan Davison, M.D.
Director of Department of Rheumatology: Harry Spier, M.D.
Affiliation: Mt. Sinai School of Medicine

Dr. Davison classifies the treatment approach here as alternative, and says that "each case is treated individually and we use all modalities available. Severe, acute cases are referred for hospitalization."

Length of treatment varies according to the patient's individual condition. The clinic handles all patients on an out-patient basis; referral for hospitalization if indicated is to Mt. Sinai. Most medical insurance plans cover the treatment at the Arthritis Clinic, and special financial arrangements are sometimes possible. These are handled by the hospital administration.

MULTIPURPOSE ARTHRITIS CENTERS
Affiliated with the National Institute of Arthritis, Diabetes, and Digestive and Kidney Diseases
National Institutes of Health
Bethesda, Md. 20205

The National Institute of Arthritis, Diabetes, and Digestive and Kidney Diseases has established, and supports, Multipurpose Arthritis Centers throughout the country. The purpose of these centers (called MACs) is two-fold: 1) to serve as major centers for research into, and to spread information on, the causes and control of arthritis and related diseases; and 2) to serve as education centers, promoting the application of available knowledge for the treatment of arthritis patients.

Each of the MACs is expected to maintain a substantial amount of ongoing basic and/or clinical research in areas related to rheumatic diseases. The funds for the various research programs are granted to the individual researcher in the particular MAC. The center funds themselves are used to support developmental and feasibility studies in rheumatological areas.

Several of the MACs are conducting clinical trials to determine whether a new medication or treatment procedure is effective in the fight against arthritis.

Another area in which the MACs serve an important function is the testing of new method of improving arthritis care at the level of the primary care physician. Some of the professional education approaches being investigated include:

- The development of a computer-based system that would enable a non-rheumatologist physician (i.e., an internist or a general practitioner) to obtain clinical consultation.
- Continuation of the Dial-Access System, by which a toll-free long-distance call connects a physician with tape-recorded information for consultation on rheumatological problems.
- Utilizing trained patient-instructors to help train medical students in the proper methods of physical examination of joints and clinical diagnosis of arthritis-related problems.

Different MACs have specific focuses; some deal primarily with lupus, others with juvenile rheumatoid arthritis, and so on. The centers share in each other's research and activities by means of annual meetings, the production of an index of the audiovisual material generated by the various centers, and other such joint ventures. The full list of the MACs follows:

University of Alabama School of Medicine, Birmingham
University of Arizona College of Medicine, Tuscon
University of California School of Medicine, San Francisco
Stanford University School of Medicine, Stanford, Calif.
University of Colorado Health Sciences Center, Denver
University of Connecticut School of Medicine, Farmington
Arthritis Center of Hawaii, Honolulu
Indiana University School of Medicine, Indianapolis
Johns Hopkins School of Medicine, Baltimore, Md.
Boston University School of Medicine, Boston, Mass.
Robert B. Brigham Hospital, Boston, Mass.
University of Michigan Medical School, Ann Arbor
University of Missouri Medical Center, Columbia
Washington University School of Medicine, St. Louis, Mo.
Dartmouth Medical School, Department of Medicine,
    Hanover, N.H.
State University of New York, Downstate Medical Center,
    Brooklyn
Cornell University Medical College, New York, N.Y.
University of Cincinnati Medical Center, Cincinnati, Ohio
Case Western Reserve University, Cleveland, Ohio
Vanderbilt University Medical Center, Nashville, Tenn.
Medical College of Wisconsin, Milwaukee

DR. CHARLES S. NEER II
161 Fort Washington Avenue
New York, N.Y. 10032
(212) 694-5528/9
Specialty: Orthopedic Surgery
Sub-specialty: Shoulder and Elbow Reconstruction
Affiliations: Columbia University College of Physicians and
              Surgeons
              New York Orthopaedic Hospital, Columbia-
              Presbyterian Medical Center

Dr. Neer classifies his approach to the treatment of arthritis as traditional and innovative. For surgical arthroplasty and total joint replacement, hospitalization lasts from two to two and a half weeks. There is a much longer period following release from the hospital during which exercises and rehabilitation occur. Dr. Neer's procedures are covered by most medical insurance plans.

DR. DAVID NEUSTADT
600 Medical Towers Building
Louisville, Ky. 40202
(502) 585-4163
Specialty: Rheumatology
Affiliation: Clinical Professor of Medicine, University of
           Louisville School of Medicine

Dr. Neustadt takes a broad approach to the treatment of arthritis, classifying it as traditional, innovative, and alternative. He states that his approach is "pending type and kind of diagnosis and stage of disease."
Length of treatment is determined on an individual basis. Hospitalization may be required. Most medical insurance plans cover Dr. Neustadt's treatment program.

NEW YORK UNIVERSITY MEDICAL CENTER
Rusk Rehabilitation Institute
400 East 34th Street
New York, N.Y. 10016
(212) 340-7300

This is one of the foremost rehabilitation centers in the country. Patients are referred by their physicians, and the staff includes specialists from the entire spectrum of rehabilitative medicine. Treatment length varies. Medical insurance plans cover most treatments.

NORTH CAROLINA BAPTIST HOSPITAL AND
   BOWMAN GRAY SCHOOL OF MEDICINE
Rheumatology Clinic
300 South Hawthorne Road
Winston-Salem, N.C. 27103
(919) 748-4209
Chief of Rheumatology: Robert A. Turner, M.D.
Director of Rheumatology Patient Care: Edward J. Pisko,
   M.D.
Affiliation: Bowman Gray School of Medicine of Wake
           Forest University

This program has been classified as traditional and innovative. The treatment program, for the most part, is traditional, with the emphasis on a multidisciplinary approach to the management of the patient. (this applies to both in- and out-patients). Emphasis is placed on the psychological impact of arthritis. All the well-established drugs that are approved for the treatment of arthritis are used.
Innovative research studies are conducted into the treatment of rheumatic diseases; some focus on psychological factors in rheumatoid arthritis. All patients who participate in experimental treatments are exempt from payment for those treatments. Most

medical insurance plans cover the non-experimental treatment program, and special financial arrangements are possible. Treatment length varies considerably. If hospitalized, a patient usually stays for only five days. Out-patients are followed for several years in most cases.

NORTHWESTERN UNIVERSITY FACULTY FOUNDATION
Arthritis Clinic
222 East Superior
Chicago, Ill. 60611
Affiliation: Northwestern University Medical School

This clinic specializes in rheumatology, orthopedic surgery, and rehabilitative medicine. It is both traditional and innovative in its approach to the treatment of arthritis. Traditional medications and methods are used to treat patients, but "innovative and experimental methods of treatment are used for those cases that are resistant to all conventional therapy."

Each patient's condition is assessed and diagnosed carefully, with an individualized treatment program designed after that. Treatment length varies, and patients whose condition requires it are hospitalized. Treatment is covered by most medical insurance plans, and special financial arrangements are possible.

DR. YUKIHIKO NOSÉ
Department of Artificial Organs
Cleveland Clinic
9500 Euclid Avenue
Cleveland, Ohio 44106
(216) 444-2470
Specialty: Artificial Organs
Affiliation: The Cleveland Clinic

Dr. Nosé is currently conducting research on cryofiltration, a form of plasmapheresis (pp. 40–41), a treatment approach he classifies as innovative. This process aids the patient by removing from the bloodstream immunocomplexes that are thought to be implicated in rheumatoid arthritis and other autoimmune diseases. Published reports of research so far show promising results.

Therapy comprises a minimum of 10 sessions, with each treatment session lasting three hours. Hospitalization is not necessary for the treatments, which generally are not covered by medical insurance plans. A patient should check with his or her insurance company to see whether coverage can be obtained.

THE OHIO PAIN AND STRESS TREATMENT CENTER
1460 West Lake Avenue
Columbus, Ohio 43221
(614) 488-5971
Director: Ivan G. Podobnikar, M.D.

Dr. Podobnikar classifies his center as innovative. There are many different modalities used in the two-week, out-patient program. Daily exercises and "swimnastics," group therapy, behavior therapy, transcutaneous electric nerve stimulations (p. 87), biofeedback training, weight and stress control, and therapeutic massage are only some of the methods employed.

Referral by a physician is not essential, but it is preferred. Each patient is carefully evaluated and examined by Dr. Podobnikar prior to admittance to the program. After completing the two-week treatment, patients continue treatment at home. There is a monthly follow-up for the first six months after the initial period.

Most medical insurance plans cover approximately 80 percent of the costs; exceptions usually include the biofeedback training and educational lectures. Requests for special financial arrangements are assessed individually, and are granted if the situation warrants.

PAIN CONTROL AND HEALTH SUPPORT SERVICES
15455 Barton Road, Suite 102B
(P.O. Box 962)
Loma Linda, Calif. 92354
(714) 796-0231
Director: Monica Neumann, M.D.
Affiliation: Loma Linda University Medical School

Dr. Neumann classifies the treatment approach here as traditional, innovative, and alternative. A wide variety of treatment modalities is offered, and if a patient has received prior therapy that was unsuccessful, methods not yet tried will be used. Such methods include transcutaneous electric nerve stimulation (p. 87), electro-acupuncture, and biofeedback. The organization does *not* provide primary care.

Patients should be referred specifically for one of the treatment programs, which include: nerve block, chronic pain syndrome, acupuncture, transcutaneous electrical neural stimulation, biofeedback, and back-care education. These programs not only treat the patient on an out-patient basis, but train the patient to continue the treatment on his or her own.

Most of the treatment modalities are covered by medical insurance plans; electro-acupuncture is an exception. Special financial arrangements can be worked out. The average length of treatment spans two to three months.

DR. ROBERT H. PERSELLIN
205 East Evergreen Street
San Antonio, Texas 78212
(512) 224-4421
Specialties: Rheumatology (Adult and Pediatric); Internal
          Medicine

Dr. Persellin classifies his approach to the treatment of arthritis as "traditional, based on current scientific information." The length of treatment varies with the degree of complexity and severity of the individual case. If indicated, hospitalization may be required. Dr. Persellin's treatment program is covered by most medical insurance plans, and special financial arrangements are possible.

DR. JAMES B. PETER
2222 Santa Monica Boulevard
Santa Monica, Calif. 90404
(213) 829-1866
Specialty: Rheumatology, Myology
Affiliations: Director, Rheumatic Disease Rehabilitation
              Program, Daniel Freeman Hospital
              Clinical Professor of Medicine and
              Rheumatology, University of California, Los
              Angeles, School of Medicine

Dr. Peter's approach to the treatment of arthritis includes education of the patient, as well as an individualized therapy program designed to meet the patient's needs.

PORTLAND NATUROPATHIC CLINIC
11231 SE Market Street
Portland, Ore. 97216
(503) 255-7355
Director: Michael Traub, N.D.
Affiliation: National College of Naturopathic Medicine
             John Bastyr College of Naturopathic Medicine
             (Seattle, Wash.)

This clinic aims to "provide complete naturopathic health care utilizing the entire realm of naturopathic therapeutics with an emphasis on treating the *whole person,* not merely the disease." The doctors are all graduates of a four-year program in medical and naturopathic sciences.

Treatment modalities include diet evaluation, fasting, nutritional supplements, hydrotherapy, physiotherapy, homeopathy, acupuncture, botanical medicine, stress reduction, counseling, and exercise. The appropriate treatment for each patient is determined after a thorough examiantion and history have been concluded; complete laboratory services are available at the clinic.

The clinic treats children as well as adults, and will work with the family of patients also. This is an out-patient clinic.

DR. CHITRANJAN S. RANAWAT
535 East 71st Street
New York, N.Y. 10021
(212) 606-1494
Specialty: Orthopedic Surgeon
Affiliations: Hospital for Special Surgery
              Cornell University Medical Center
              New York Hospital

Dr. Ranawat specializes in the reconstructive surgery for rheumatoid arthritis and osteoarthritis, and classifies his treatment approach as innovative. The average length of hospitalization for such surgery is 12 days. There is, of course, a period of time after surgery during which exercising and rehabilitation are essential.

Most medical insurance plans cover these procedures, but no special financial arrangements are possible.

REHABILITATION INSTITUTE OF CHICAGO
345 East Superior Street
Chicago, Ill. 60611
(312) 649-6066
Director of Physiatry: Judith Sutin, M.D.
Directors of Rheumatology: Roland Chang, M.D.; Frank
Schmid, M.D.
Affiliations: Northwestern University Medical School
Northwestern McGaw Medical Center
The institute's program has been classified as innovative in its approach to the treatment of arthritis. The stated purpose of the Arthritis Rehabilitation Unit is "to help patients with disabling polyarticular disease maximize functional potential and quality of life within the constraints of their process."

Treatment length varies; hospitalization is usually three to five weeks in duration. Out-patient status during treatment is possible as well. Most medical insurance plans cover treatment here, and special financial arrangements are possible.

DR. EMMANUEL RUDD
One West 64th Street
New York, N.Y. 10023
(212) 877-2236
Specialty: Rheumatology
Affiliations: Hospital for Special Surgery
New York Hospital
Cornell University Medical College
Dr. Rudd classifies his approach to treatment as traditional. The program he prescribes depends on the patient's needs. Medication and home exercise and joint protection are at the core of the treatment. Orthopedic surgery and post-operative rehabilitation may be required.

On occasion Dr. Rudd has to hospitalize a patient during the diagnostic process. This happens if more extensive testing is required in order to arrive at a proper diagnosis.

ST. JOSEPH CLINIC
2900 North Lake Shore Drive
Chicago, Ill. 60657
(312) 975-3080
St. Joseph's is a pain control clinic. Its program entails a variety of modalities, including nutrition therapy, occupational therapy, psychological counseling, and transcutaneous electric nerve stimulation (p. 87).

ST. MARY'S HOSPITAL
Pain Management Center
Rochester, Minn. 55901
(507) 285-5921
Director of Center: Toshihiko Maruta, M.D.
Affiliations: Mayo Medical School
Mayo Graduate School of Medicine
Patients are admitted to the Pain Management Center after a complete evaluation by Mayo Clinic physicians. The Center is

operated jointly by the Mayo Clinic and St. Mary's Hospital. Its approach, according to Dr. Maruta, is alternative. It is for patients with prolonged, treatment-resistant pain. The center's staff comprises a psychiatrist, a clinical psychologist, a program coordinator, an occupational therapist, and nursing personnel. Specialists in all the medical and surgical fields are available from the Mayo Clinic for consultation.

The program is "intended to help the patient cope with pain more effectively, to decrease disability, and to increase self-management of the pain problem." Such modalities as rehabilitation medicine, behavior modification, education, biofeedback techniques, and counseling are used, depending on each patient's need. The main phase of treatment "emphasizes techniques which reduce use of medications and complaints of pain while increasing physical activity and independent functioning."

The center employs a specially designed medication-reduction technique, and offers individualized activity programs tailored to the specific patient. The final phase of the treatment involves family members in counseling, and usually lasts about three days.

The total length of the program is approximately three weeks, all on an in-patient basis. Most medical insurance plans cover treatment in this program. No special financial arrangements are available.

DR. PETER SCHUR
Robert B. Bingham Division
Brigham and Women's Hospital
75 Francis Street
Boston, Mass. 02115
(617) 732-5350
Specialty: Rheumatology (Lupus)

Dr. Schur treats lupus patients and is also a grant recipient of NIADDK (p. 67). His research programs have included the investigation of several immunologic antigen-antibody reaction tests that have been developed for lupus, the investigation of genetic markers in a form of juvenile arthritis, and investigations into the white cell activity (or lack of activity) in immune responses in lupus patients.

DR. ROBERT SIFFERT
Mt. Sinai School of Medicine
Mt. Sinai Medical Center
Fifth Avenue and 100th Street
New York, N.Y. 10029
(212) 876-2111
Specialty: Orthopedics
Affiliation: Professor/Chairman of Orthopedics,
          Mt. Sinai School of Medicine

Dr. Siffert classifies his approach as traditional. It involves surgical treatment of arthritis damage. The process of joint replacement, from diagnosis through rehabilitation, takes an average of three months, although the hospitalization stage lasts only two weeks.

Treatment is covered by most medical insurance plans, but no special financial arrangements are possible.

DR. JAMES W. SMITH
Cleveland Clinic
9500 Euclid Avenue
Cleveland, Ohio 44106
(216) 444-2470
Specialty: Plasmapheresis
Affiliation: The Cleveland Clinic Foundation

Dr. Smith is the head of the clinical membrane plasmapheresis research program, a treatment approach he classifies as "innovative." The program currently under investigation concerns cryofiltration (p. 41), a form of plasmapheresis. This procedure is not covered by most medical insurance plans; patients have to discuss coverage on a case-by-case basis with their insurance carrier. Special financial arrangements are possible.

SPAIN REHABILITATION CENTER
171 Sixth Avenue South
Birmingham, Ala. 35205
(205) 934-2130
Affiliation: University of Alabama, Birmingham

The center's specialties are rheumatology and rehabilitation medicine. Tratment is described as empirical and conservative.

Length of treatment varies. Most patients are seen on an out-patient basis, but hospitalization, if necessary, usually lasts about 10 days. Most medical insurance plans cover treatment at the center, and special financial arrangements are possible.

STANFORD UNIVERSITY HOSPITAL
Stanford Immunology Clinic
Stanford University,
Stanford, Calif. 94305
(415) 497-6001
Director: James F. Fries, M.D.
Affiliation: Stanford University

Dr. Fries classifies the treatment approach at this clinic as both traditional and innovative. It follows "rigorous scientific medicine," incorporating a multidisciplinary approach that includes medication, surgery, exercise, and education. The clinic is a national focus for patient education programs about arthritis.

At the same time that it follows a traditional program, the clinic is also involved in a "systematic evaluation of new drugs and treatment modalities," one of which is total nodal irradiation (also called "total lymphoid irradiation," p. 68). Selected patients are treated with experimental protocols.

Usually only patients with difficult and complex problems are accepted from physician referrals. Length of treatment depends on the patient's problem; most patients are seen on an out-patient basis. Most medical insurance plans cover treatment here. No special financial arrangements are available.

STATE UNIVERSITY HOSPITAL
Arthritis Clinic
Downstate Medical Center
470 Clarkson Avenue
Brooklyn, N.Y. 11203
(212) 270-1321
Director of Clinic: Charles R. Steinman, M.D.
Affiliation: State University of New York, Downstate
    Medical Center

This clinic follows a traditional approach to the treatment of arthritis. Patients are seen on either an in- or an out-patient basis. There are about 75 patients per clinic session.

Most medical insurance plans cover treatment at the clinic, and special financial arrangements can be worked out.

DR. ALFRED D. STEINBERG
Building 10, Room 9N 218
National Institutes of Health
Bethesda, Md. 20014
(301) 496-3374
Specialty: Rheumatology
Affiliation: National Institutes of Health (National Institute
    of Arthritis, Diabetes, and Digestive and
    Kidney Diseases: NIADDK)

Dr. Steinberg classifies his approach to the treatment of arthritis as innovative. Treatment by Dr. Steinberg himself is limited to patients whose particular conditions fit the research needs of the particular project on which he is currently working. All patients who end up as part of the studies at NIADDK (or any branch of the NIH) must be referred by their physician. Each case is considered carefully to see if it fits the project's need. Patients are treated at the Warren G. Magnuson Clinical Center in Bethesda, free of charge.

DR. ROBERT L. SWEZEY
Suite 223
2200 Santa Monica Boulevard
Santa Monica, Calif. 90404
(213) 829-7926
Specialties: Internal Medicine; Rheumatology; Physical
    Medicine and Rehabilitation
Affiliations: Medical Director, The Arthritis and Back Pain
    Center, Inc.
    University of California, Los Angeles

Dr. Swezey classifies his treatment approach as traditional and innovative. Diagnostic methods and pharmacological therapies for rheumatic diseases are conventional. What Dr. Swezey feels is innovative about his treatment is that it emphasizes patient education and integrated rehabilitation therapies, including occupational therapy, physical therapy, andpsychological counseling. The entire program is available to the patient in one out-patient setting.

Dr. Swezey and his staff have designed programs especially for a variety of rheumatological disorders. Hospitalization may be involved as part of the therapy. The program is acceptable to most medical insurance plans, although no special financial arrangements can be made.

TEXAS CHILDREN'S HOSPITAL
Department of Rheumatology
P.O. Box 20269
Houston, Texas 77030
(713) 791-3134
Director of Department: Earl J. Brewer, Jr., M.D.
Affiliation: Baylor College of Medicine, Department of
            Pediatrics

The treatment approach here is both traditional and innovative. Treatment varies according to the patient's needs. There are from five to 15 children hospitalized at any given time, and patient visits number from 50 to 80 a week.

Treatment here is covered by most medical insurance plans, and special financial arrangements can be worked out.

DR. CHARLES TOURTELOTTE
Temple University Hospital
3401 North Broad Street
Philadelphia, Pa. 19140
(215) 221-3606
Specialties: Internal Medicine; Rheumatology
Affiliations: Temple University School of Medicine and
             Hospital (Arthritis Clinic, Rehabilitation Unit,
             Out-Patient Unit)
             Milville (N.J.) Hospital (Arthritis Clinic)

Dr. Tourtelotte classifies his approach to the treatment of arthritis as "comprehensive traditional." He adds that "it is comprehensive with consideration of all aspects of the patient's condition and environmental circumstances in diagnosis and management." The length of treatment varies according to the patient's condition.

Dr. Tourtelotte's treatment program is covered by most medical insurance plans, and special financial arrangements are possible.

UNIVERSITY OF ALABAMA, BIRMINGHAM
University Station
Birmingham, Ala. 35294
(205) 934-5306
Head of Clinic: William J. Koopman, M.D.
Affiliations: University of Alabama (Birmingham,
             Huntsville, and Tuscaloosa campuses)

The approach to the treatment of arthritis here is innovative. A multidisciplinary team approach is used, with doctors from various specialties in consultation.

Treatment is on an in-patient basis, and the average length of treatment varies according to the patient's condition. Medical insurance plans cover treatment here, and special financial arrangements are possible.

UNIVERSITY OF ALABAMA-BIRMINGHAM MEDICAL CENTER

Pain Management Center
1920 Seventh Avenue, South
Birmingham, Ala. 35233
(205) 934-6174
Head of Department: H. Ronald Vinik, M.D.
Affiliation: University of Alabama, Birmingham

Dr. Vinik classifies the center's treatment approach as traditional; the center coordinates physical therapy, psychological treatment, and nerve blocks with treatment provided at the university's arthritis clinic.

Length of treatment varies according to the patient's condition; the center sees patients on both an in- and an out-patient basis. Treatment here is covered by most medical insurance plans, and special financial arrangements are possible.

UNIVERSITY OF CALIFORNIA, LOS ANGELES, SCHOOL OF MEDICINE

Pain Management Center
Department of Anesthesiology
10833 La Conte Avenue
Los Angeles, Calif. 90024
(213) 825-4291
Director: Richard Kroening, M.D.
Affiliation: University of California, Los Angeles

The treatment approach here is described as traditional, innovative, and alternative. It is a multi-modal program, with each patient's needs evaluated individually. Patients must be referred by either a doctor or a psychologist before the evaluation process can begin. Psychological as well as physical aspects of the case are considered.

Among the procedures employed as part of the treatment program are regional anesthesia, transcutaneous electrical neural stimulation (p. 87), acupuncture, physical therapy, medication tailoring and detoxification, individual psychotherapy and behavior modification, relaxation and self-hypnosis training, biofeedback, and structured pain-management classes.

Treatment is covered by most medical insurance plans, although Medicare covers only some of the procedures. It is best to check with your insurance carrier to find out. No special financial arrangements are possible. All treatment is on an out-patient basis.

UNIVERSITY OF CINCINNATI MEDICAL CENTER

Pain Control Center
234 Goodman Street
Old Administration Building
Cincinnati, Ohio 45267
(Mailing address: University of Cincinnati, ML#586)
(513) 872-5664
Head of Center: P. Prithvi Raj, M.D.

This program is classified as innovative in its treatment approach. The aim of the therapy at this center is to enable the patient to "reduce medication and to lead a more active and productive life." The patients accepted to the program have to be referred by their physicians (written referral is necessary). The evaluation process determines the individual treatment plan for each patient.

Various procedures are employed, including sympathetic nerve blocks, peripheral nerve blocks, acupuncture, and transcutaneous electrical neural stimulation (p. 87). Treatment takes place over a three month period, in most cases. The emphasis is on out-patient treatment, although there may be as many as four in-patients a week. Treatment is covered by most medical insurance plans, and special financial arrangements can be made.

UNIVERSITY OF CONNECTICUT HEALTH CENTER
Division of Rheumatic Diseases
Farmington, Conn. 06032
(203) 674-2160/2911

The treatment approach here is both traditional and innovative. After an exact diagnosis is arrived at, using standard methods, conventional treatment is begun. If that fails, experimental treatment is used.

Length of treatment depends on the form and severity of the patient's disease. Hospitalization is part of the program if needed. Treatment is covered by most medical insurance plans, and special financial arrangements are possible.

UNIVERSITY OF IOWA HOSPITALS AND CLINICS
Rheumatology Clinic
Iowa City, Iowa 52240
(319) 356-2413
Director: R.F. Ashman, M.D.
Affiliation: University of Iowa College of Medicine

The treatment approach at the Rheumatology Clinic is both traditional and innovative. The conventional therapeutic measures are employed, but new experimental drugs and procedures are offered to "appropriate patients on clinical research projects." The Arthritis Care Team is a multidisciplinary unit providing a wide range of therapies and services.

Patients are seen on both an in- and an out-patient basis, with approximately 100 out-patients treated each week. Treatment in the clinic is covered by most medical insurance plans, and special financial arrangements can be worked out.

UNIVERSITY OF MICHIGAN
Arthritis Clinic
Arthritis In-Patient Clinic
Lupus Clinic
Ann Arbor, Mich. 48109
(313) 764-4186
Affiliation: University of Michigan Medical School

The treatment approaches in these three clinics are traditional and innovative. The program has been summarized as follows: "Multispecialty teams provide appropriate rheumatic disease therapy after a thorough history, physical examination, and indicated X-rays and laboratory tests are performed."

Most patients are seen as out-patients. Treatment length varies. Most medical insurance plans cover treatment at these clinics, and special financial arrangements are possible.

UNIVERSITY OF MINNESOTA
Arthritis Clinics
Department of Medicine
Box 108, Mayo Memorial Building
420 Delaware Street, S.E.
Minneapolis, Minn. 55455
(612) 376-8613
Director, Section of Rheumatology: Ronald P. Messner,
M.D.
Affiliation: University of Minnesota Medical School

Treatment at the Arthritis Clinics is classified as traditional. The clinics function primarily as referral centers for difficult cases. Although referral by a physician is common, it is not necessary; patients may make appointments directly. The most important part of the entire procedure is to establish the proper diagnosis. In most cases this is accomplished through out-patient visits, but in some cases a short hospital stay may be necessary.

Treatment programs are communicated to the patient's doctor, if that patient lives outside the area. That doctor then becomes the primary care physician; in such cases, the patient usually returns to the clinics for check-ups or for a re-evaluation. Patients who live in the area may either continue at the clinics, as out-patients, or receive their primary care from their own physician.

Treatment is covered by most medical insurance plans, and special financial arrangements are possible.

UNIVERSITY OF NEBRASKA HOSPITAL AND CLINIC
Nebraska Pain Management Center
42nd and Dewey Avenue
Omaha, Neb. 68105
(402) 559-4364
Medical Director: F. Miles Skultety, M.D.
Affiliation: University of Nebraska Medical Center

The treatment approach here includes many innovative modalities, among which are biofeedback and relaxation techniques. The treatment program lasts four weeks. All patients are seen on an in-patient basis. Treatment is covered by most medical insurance plans.

UNIVERSITY OF NORTH CAROLINA SCHOOL OF MEDICINE
Arthritis Clinic
Division of Rheumatology and Immunology
Department of Medicine
932 Faculty Laboratory Office Building 231 H
Chapel Hill, N.C. 27514
(919) 966-4191
Chief, Division of Rheumatology: John B. Winfield, M.D.
Clinic Director: William J. Yount, M.D.

The treatment approach of this arthritis clinic is classified as innovative. The Division of Rheumatology and Immunology is the recipient of a grant from NIADDK (p. 67), and is a multipurpose arthritis center "for the comprehensive approach as well as innovative approaches for patients with all types of arthritis." Treatment length varies with the type of arthritis, but "an effort is made to provide a comprehensive program of long-term management." Patients are seen on both an in- and an out-patient basis; there is an in-patient rehabilitation unit available for intensive rehabilitation efforts.

The Division of Rheumatology and Immunology also has a "strong committment to both clinical and basic research in the rheumatic diseases as well as evaluation of new forms of therapy. . . ."

Treatment is covered by most medical insurance plans, and special financial arrangements can be worked out.

UNIVERSITY OF VIRGINIA MEDICAL CENTER
Department of Anesthesiology Pain Clinic
Box 293
Charlottesville, Va. 22908
(804) 924-5581
Director: John C. Rowlingson, M.D.
Affiliation: University of Virginia School of Medicine

This clinic's treatment approach is classified as alternative. Treatment is varied, and includes elimination of dependence on habituation drugs, exercise and activity programs, relaxation training, nerve blocks, transcutaneous electrical neutral stimulation (p. 87), biofeedback, and temperature training biofeedback. There are also various forms of psychological support programs.

Treatment length varies. Most medical insurance plans cover the treatment program, and special financial arrangements are possible.

UNIVERSITY OF WASHINGTON MEDICAL SCHOOL
Clinical Pain Service
Northeast Pacific
Seattle, Wash. 98195
(206) 543-3200

This pain service has been classified as traditional, innovative, and alternative. It offers a multidisciplinary approach to the treatment of chronic pain. Patients must be referred by a physician in order to be evaluated. Not all patients who are evaluated are accepted into the program; once evaluated, however, a patient will be advised by the service as to the "most likely choices for diagnosis and treatment."

Individuals accepted into the program have access to a full range of modalities; each patient's program is based on his or her condition and needs. Treatment length varies, and patients are seen on both an in-and an out-patient basis. Treatment is covered by most medical insurance plans.

VETERANS ADMINISTRATION HOSPITAL
Arthritis Clinic
North Heartland
White River Junction, Vt. 05001
(802) 295-9363
Chief of Rheumatology: Thomas H. Taylor, M.D.
Affiliation: Dartmouth Medical School

This clinic has a traditional approach to the treatment of arthritis. Medications, physical and occupational therapies, and orthopedic services are all individualized to the patient's disease and condition. Patients are seen on both an in- and an out-patient basis, and treatment length varies.

Most medical insurance plans cover treatment at this clinic; no special financial arrangements are available.

WEST VIRGINIA UNIVERSITY MEDICAL CENTER
Rheumatology Clinic
Morgantown, W. Va. 26506
(304) 293-4901
Head of Clinic: Anthony G. Di Bartolomeo, M.D.
Affiliation: West Virginia University

This clinic applies an innovative approach to the treatment of arthritis. A full range of drugs is employed, with choice of medication determined by the patient's condition. All patients are seen as out-patients. Most medical insurance plans cover treatment here, and special financial arrangements can be made.

DR. ROBERT F. WILLKENS
Harborview Medical Center
325 Ninth Avenue
Seattle, Wash. 98104
(206) 223-3156
Specialties: Internal Medicine; Rheumatology
Affiliations: Head of Arthritis Division, Harborview Medical
            Center
            University of Washington

Dr. Willkens has classified his approach to arthritis treatment as traditional and alternative. He says that "arthritis is thought to be caused by a disorder in the body's immune system, which results in an attack on the lining of the joints."He has substituted new drugs in the treatment of arthritis. Prostaglandin inhibitors are used to reduce pain instead of aspirin; gold pills taken orally are prescribed rather than injections of gold salts.

Treatment length varies according to the patient's condition; hospitalization is occasionally required. Treatment is covered by most medical insurance plans, and special financial arrangements are possible.

DR. COLIN H. WILSON, JR.
Emory University School of Medicine
69 Butler Street, S.E.
Atlanta, Ga. 30303
(404) 588-3640
Specialties: Rheumatology; Immunology
Affiliations: Emory University School of Medicine: Director,
Division of Rheumatology-Immunology;
Professor of Medicine (Rheumatology-
Immunology); Associate Professor of Physical
Medicine and Rehabilitation

Dr. Wilson classifies his approach to the treatment of arthritis as traditional. His treatment does not include hospitalization. It is covered by most medical insurance plans, and special financial arrangements are possible.

DR. MORRIS ZIFF
Department of Internal Medicine
University of Texas Health Science Center
5323 Harry Hines Boulevard
Dallas, Texas 75235
(214) 688-3466
Specialties: Internal Medicine; Rheumatology
Affiliations: University of Texas Health Science Center at
Dallas
Parkland Memorial Hospital

Dr. Ziff classifies his approach to the treatment of arthritis as traditional. Treatment is usually long-term. Hospitalization is part of the program if needed. Treatment is covered by most medical insurance plans.

DR. NATHAN ZVAIFLER
University of California Medical Center
225 Dickinson Street
San Diego, Calif. 92103
(619) 294-5982
Specialties: Internal Medicine; Rheumatology
Affiliation: University of California Medical Center, San
Diego

Dr. Zvaifler classifies his approach to the treatment of arthritis as traditional. Hospitalization may be required, depending upon the individual patient. Dr. Zvaifler's treatment program is covered by most medical insurance plans, but no special financial arrangements are available.

7

PROFESSIONAL ASSOCIATIONS, FOUNDATIONS, ORGANIZATIONS, AND SELF-HELP GROUPS

The various institutions and organizations in this chapter all have a common purpose: serving the different components of the rheumatic disease "audience." By "audience" we mean not only those who are afflicted, but also the families of patients, and health professionals of any persuasion. By disseminating information, providing research funds, and/or making available a variety of services, the groups listed here help to heighten our awareness of the diseases, the available therapies, and the promise of help and hope.

The sole public function of some of these groups is to provide referral lists of specialists in a particular medical approach or area of practice. Such groups serve their members in many other ways, including the sponsorship of symposia that allow exchange of research information. Other groups are focused on the public's need for information concerning ways to ameliorate the variety of problems caused by a disease.

Whatever the group and its audience, together they form a support network for anyone whose life has been, or might be, affected in any way by rheumatic disease.

Information in the following entries comes, for the most part, from questionnaires sent to the groups. There are some listings for groups and associations that did not return their questionnaires; these warrant inclusion for the referral function they can serve to both the professional world and the public.

PROFESSIONAL ASSOCIATIONS

AMERICAN ACADEMY OF OSTEOPATHY
12 West Locust Street
P.O. Box 750
Newark, Ohio 43055
(614) 349-8701

This is the national membership headquarters; AAO has more than 20 state and local groups. It conducts graduate courses and has a library of works on osteopathy. The group publishes a quarterly newsletter and an annual directory of its members. Lists of Doctors of Osteopathy in different states can be obtained from the academy.

AMERICAN ACADEMY OF PHYSICAL MEDICINE AND REHABILITATION
30 North Michigan Avenue
Chicago, Ill. 60602
(312) 236-9512

This professional organization sponsors conventions, symposia, and publications for those involved in the areas of physical medicine and rehabilitation. Lists of specialists in different states can be obtained from the academy.

AMERICAN ASSOCIATION OF HOMES FOR THE AGING
Suite 770
1050 17th Street, N.W.
Washington, D.C. 20036
(202) 296-5960
Director: Sheldon L. Goldberg

This is a national organization of facilities for the aged. The primary goal of this group is "to aid and assist our member facilities with health care and housing services for residents of the home; [and] to provide educational services and planning for the future."

If you are considering placing a relative in such a home, check with AAHA to find out if the home you are considering is a member; membership does ensure a certain level of care, although it is no guarantee of the suitability of a home for your needs.

Member facilities pay an annual fee which is dependent on the size of the facility.

AMERICAN CHIROPRACTIC ASSOCIATION
1916 Wilson Boulevard
Arlington, Va. 22201
(703) 276-8800

This is a professional association. It is active in promoting chiropractic medicine and gaining acceptance for its practice. ACA publishes a monthly journal, a bimonthly magazine, and an annual directory. It also sponsors a national convention.

AMERICAN COLLEGE OF PREVENTIVE MEDICINE
Suite 403
1015 15th Street, N.W.
Washington, D.C. 20005
(202) 789-0003

This professional organization has as its members those specialists who are engaged in the practice and teaching of, and research in, preventive medicine. Information is shared through national conventions, a bimonthly newsletter, symposia, and regional meetings. Lists of specialists may be obtained from this office.

AMERICAN COLLEGE OF RADIOLOGY
20 North Wacker Drive
Chicago, Ill. 60606
(312) 236-4963

This organization is of and for radiology professionals. More than 50 state groups are affiliated with ACR. Through symposia, an annual convention, and various publications (including a monthly newsletter), information is shared on the newest advances in the specialty. ACR sponsors research in this specialty and its applications.

Information about the various state groups (and specialists in the different states) can be obtained from this office.

AMERICAN HOLISTIC HEALTH SCIENCES ASSOCIATION
Suite 208
1766 Cumberland Green
St. Charles, Ill. 60174
(312) 377-1929

This organization accepts as members health practitioners, consultants, counselors, and health students of the various therapies that constitute holistic treatment. Some of these are: acupuncture, chiropractic, naturopath, reflexology, shiatsu, nutrition, homeopathy, and psychology. The group seeks to share data on treatments and remedies among its members, as well as to educate the public in the holistic approach to health care.

Among the group's activities are meetings and the publication of a bibliography and a newsletter (p. 136).

AMERICAN MEDICAL ASSOCIATION
535 North Dearborn Street
Chicago, Ill. 60610
(312) 751-6000

This is the predominant medical association in the United States, in terms of both membership and power. It has more than 56 state and regional groups and almost 2,000 county medical societies. Its approach to the treatment of rheumatic diseases is traditional.

AMA's functions relate to different "audiences": The public is served by the dissemination of scientific information, and by the association's participation in establishing standards for medical training and hospitals. The medical profession benefits from the dissemination of scientific information and by AMA's advocacy position in legislative issues on both the state and federal levels. Individual doctors are aided by the association's physicians placement service and by its practice-management counseling service. AMA also publishes a weekly newsletter (p. 135) and journal.

AMERICAN OCCUPATIONAL THERAPY ASSOCIATION
1383 Piccard Drive
Rockville, Md. 20815
(301) 948-9626
Executive Director: James J. Garibaldi
President: Robert K. Bing

This is a national professional organization of registered occupational therapists and registered and certified occupational therapy assistants. The members of this association provide "services to people whose lives have been disrupted by physical injury or illness . . . [or] the aging process." Information on the functions of an occupational therapist is exchanged through meetings and conventions, symposia, and publications.

Membership in the association is a guarantee of the therapist's certification; lists of such individuals are available through this office.

AMERICAN ORTHOPAEDIC ASSOCIATION
444 North Michigan Avenue
Chicago, Ill. 60611
(312) 822-0979

This group is a professional society of bone and joint surgeons. Anyone interested in finding a specialist can obtain names of members from this office. The group publishes a journal throughout the year and a newsletter every four months. It has an annual convention at which information about new advances is shared.

AMERICAN OSTEOPATHIC ASSOCIATION
212 East Ohio Street
Chicago, Ill. 60611
(312) 280-5800

As a professional association, AOA serves to support the spreading and sharing of information about this medical system. It has more than 50 state groups and 200 local chapters. Members are osteopathic physicians, surgeons, and graduates of approved osteopathic colleges.

AOA inspects and accredits osteopathic colleges; certifies specialists; sponsors a national board of examiners that meets most state licensing requirements; and maintains a compulsory continuing education program in medicine for its members.

The association also funds research at osteopathic colleges and hospitals, awards scholarships, and maintains a media center on osteopathic medicine. Names of Doctors of Osteopathy in different states may be obtained from the state or local chapters, whose addresses are available from this office.
AOA publishes a monthly journal (p. 134).

AMERICAN OSTEOPATHIC COLLEGE OF RHEUMATOLOGY
201 Homestead Avenue
Maybrook, N.Y. 12543
(914) 628-8363

This is a professional organization of Doctors of Osteopathy who specialize in the treatment of the rheumatic diseases. It sponsors conventions, and maintains a directory of its members.

AMERICAN RHEUMATISM ASSOCIATION
1314 Spring Street
Atlanta, Ga. 30309
(404) 872-7100, ext. 209
Executive Director: Lynn Bonfiglio

This association is the medical section of the Arthritis Foundation (p. 127). Its membership is composed of doctors, scientists, and others who share a common interest in the various rheumatic diseases. ARA sponsors research and promotes the training and teaching of physicians in the care of patients with these diseases.
The association publishes a monthly journal and a biennial review. It holds national conventions, where workshops and discussion groups serve as a means of disseminating new findings.

AMERICAN SOCIETY FOR CLINICAL NUTRITION
9650 Rockville Pike
Bethesda, Md. 20014
(301) 530-7110

This society is composed of doctors and scientists who work in or have an interest in clinical nutrition research. Its aim is to encourage and promote teaching, research, and the publication of progress in this specialty. ASCN publishes a monthly journal (p. 134) and has an annual convention.

HOMEOPATHIC FOUNDATION
3 East 85th Street
New York, N.Y. 10028
(212) 288-0758

This foundation is composed of homeopathic physicians who are combining their efforts in research in homeopathic medicine. The group maintains a library of works on homeopathy, and holds a convention annually.

INTERNATIONAL CHIROPRACTORS ASSOCIATION
Suite 800
1901 L Stieet, N.W.
Washington, D.C. 20036
(202) 659-6476

This professional organization has more than 5,000 members. Among other activities, it supports the continuing education of its members, maintains a library, sponsors committees that monitor the profession of chiropractic medicine, publishes several newsletters, reviews, and a directory, and sponsors an annual convention. Anyone interested in chiropractic can obtain information from this group.

NATIONAL ASSOCIATION FOR HOME CARE
519 C Street, N.E.
Washington D.C. 20002
(202) 547-7424
President: Val J. Halamandaris

This national organization represents home care professionals and paraprofessionals. It aims to provide educational and legislative regulatory advocacy for the nation's home health care agencies, hospices, and homemaker/home health aide organizations.

Membership in this association is an indication that the member facility or organization subscribes to the standards set by the national group. Information on a service or facility could be corroborated through this office.

NAHC publishes a newsletter in conjunction with the National Homecaring Council in New York (p. 126), and a monthly magazine, *Caring*, which is distributed free to members and costs $36 a year for non-members.

NATIONAL COLLEGE OF NATUROPATHIC MEDICINE
11231 S. E. Market Street
Portland, Ore. 97216
(503) 255-4860

This is the only college for naturopathic medicine in the United States. It is included in this list of organizations because the college, through its library and administrative offices, can serve as a source of information on naturopathic medicine, on organizations that practice naturopathy, and on practitioners themselves. The college grants a four-year N.D. degree. Naturopathic physicians are licensed in eight states at present: Arizona, Connecticut, Florida, Hawaii, Nevada, Oregon, Utah, and Washington.

NATIONAL GERIATRICS SOCIETY
212 West Wisconsin Avenue,
Milwaukee, Wis. 53202
(414) 272-4130

This is an organization of institutions that provide long-term care and treatment of chronically ill elderly people. The society promotes standards for proper operation and administration of such facilities. It acts as a consultant to its member institutions, helping them solve problems and establish geriatric programs. This group also seeks to expand public awareness of these programs.

NATIONAL HOMECARING COUNCIL
235 Park Avenue South
New York, N.Y. 10003
(212) 674-4990
Director: Florence M. Moore

This national, non-profit organization aims to promote the development of quality homemaker/home health aide service. The NHC sets standards for member agencies, operates an accreditation program, prepares basic training materials, and conducts meetings and seminars on homecare topics and problems.

Those seeking homemaker/home health aide services can call on NHC's information and referral service; the same service also helps members seeking work. Another of its functions is to prepare materials for the consumer (see Chapter 6, *Publications*).

NATIONAL INSTITUTE OF ARTHRITIS, DIABETES,
    AND DIGESTIVE AND KIDNEY DISEASES
National Institutes of Health
Bethesda, Md. 20205
Director: Lester B. Salans, M.D.

This division of the National Institutes of Health serves many functions. It is a source of research funds (p. 67), the impetus behind the creation of Multipurpose Arthritis Centers across the country (p. 103), and the resource behind the Arthritis Information Clearinghouse (p. 147).

NIADDK comprises two divisions: the extramural division is in charge of all programs that are funded by NIADDK but are conducted at other facilities; the intramural division conducts clinical and laboratory investigations within the institute's own facilities. NIADDK sponsors symposia, workshops, and publications about its work and that of its grant recipients.

The extramural division's director is Dr. Lawrence E. Shulman, Director of Arthritis, Musculoskeletal, and Skin Diseases (Building 31, Room 9A35). Dr. Henry Metzger is the Director of the Division of Arthritis and Rheumatism (the intramural section: Building 10, Room 9N222).

NATIONAL REHABILITATION ASSOCIATION
633 South Washington Street
Alexandria, Va. 22314
(703) 836-0850

This group serves professionals who are interested in the rehabilitation of the physically handicapped. Among its members are physicians, therapists of all kinds, counselors, and other practitioners whose work relates to rehabilitation.

NRA publishes a bimonthly newsletter and a quarterly journal. It also sponsors an annual convention, at which workshops and discussions are held to disseminate innovations and research findings.

SOCIETY FOR CLINICAL ECOLOGY
Suite 490
2005 Franklin Street
Denver, Colo. 80205
(303) 622-9755
President: Francis J. Waickman, M.D.
Secretary: Del Stigler, M.D.

This is a national organization whose members are clinical ecologists (pp. 49–51). The society offers a physician referral service. It sponsors seminars and meetings, including a national convention, aimed at broadening awareness of clinical ecology and its applications.

The society's publications include a textbook; a directory that lists not only the members but also the types of procedures each employs; a quarterly newsletter (p. 139); a program syllabus containing abstracts and some complete presentations from the advanced seminars the group holds; and archives of early material about clinical ecology and case studies. The society also has tapes of various proceedings, and supports an educational fund.

FOUNDATIONS, ORGANIZATIONS, AND SELF-HELP GROUPS

AMERICAN FOUNDATION FOR HOMEOPATHY
7297-H Lee Highway
Falls Church Va. 22042

This is a philanthropic, non-profit organization. Its purpose is to assist other homeopathic groups in research and educational programs. It raises funds and provides consultation services to that end.

It is a good source of names and addresses of other groups and associations dedicated to the study and practice of homeopathy.

ARTHRITIS FOUNDATION
1314 Spring Street
Atlanta, Ga. 30309
Director: Clifford M. Clarke

This is a national organization, with 71 chapters—at least one in all states but Alaska. The foundation also has branch offices; these combined with the state groups total 150 offices.

The purpose of the Arthritis Foundation is "to find the cause and cure for the many forms of arthritis; to create public understanding of these diseases; [and] to provide services to patients, serve as patient advocate and . . . combat unproven remedies." The foundation sponsors education clubs, exercise classes and swim therapy programs, patient counseling services and referral services, public education programs, government advocacy at both the state and the national level, education programs for health professionals, and a home assessment program for patients' use in adapting their residences to meet their needs.

Some of these programs are organized and implemented by the local chapters and others are directed from the national office. The Atlanta office serves as both national and Atlanta headquarters.

The Arthritis Foundation supports a conservative approach to the treatment of the rheumatic diseases. It is very careful to warn the public of what it believes are useless treatment modalities.

The foundation has several publications, including a quarterly newsletter (p. 137).

ARTHRITIS PATIENTS ASSOCIATION
c/o Robert Bingham, M.D.
1000 South Anaheim Boulevard, Suite 301
Anaheim, Calif. 92805
(714) 776-3222

This is a patients' group for those who believe in natural therapies for the treatment of arthritis. It is affiliated with the Desert Arthritis Medical Clinic under the direction of Dr. Robert Bingham. Members have an interest in a treatment plan that relieves the various rheumatic diseases without relying on drugs on surgery.

ASSOCIATION FOR THE CARE OF CHILDREN'S HEALTH
3615 Wisconsin Avenue
Washington, D.C. 20016
Executive Director: Beverley H. Johnson

This is a multidisciplinary organization that focuses on the emotional and developmental needs of children and their families in all types of health care situations. It strives to improve the quality of health care. A national organization, it has approximately 3,500 members, with 45 regional affiliate chapters in the United States and Canada.

ACCH publishes a variety of pamphlets and other works (see Chapter 8, *Publications*). It sponsors a national conference, regional institutes, and local meetings. It also coordinates a nationwide public education campaign called "Children and Hospitals Week," the purpose of which is to alert the public to the needs of children with health problems.

CHILDREN IN HOSPITALS
31 Wilshire Park
Needham, Mass. 02192

This is a regional organization, serving the state of Massachusetts and, in particular, the Boston area. It is a non-profit group, consisting of parents and health care professionals who seek to educate all those concerned about the needs of children and parents for continued and ample contact when either is hospitalized. The organization encourages hospitals to adopt flexible visiting policies and to provide living-in accommodations whenever possible.

CIH is staffed entirely by volunteers; it offers personal counseling, sends speakers to various interested groups, publishes a newsletter, has a set of guidelines for parents, and offers a bibliography of books, films, and appropriate play materials for children facing hospitalization.

CLINICAL ECOLOGY ASSOCIATION OF SOUTHERN CALIFORNIA
17400 West Irvine Boulevard
Tustin, Calif. 92680

This is a group of patients who have suffered from various ecologic diseases and/or whose physical and mental health has improved through treatment with clinical ecology techniques.

ENVIRONMENTAL ILLNESS ASSOCIATION OF NORTHERN CALIFORNIA
Oakland, Calif.
(415) 444-5723

This, like the Clinical Ecology Association of Southern California, is a group of patients whose illness has been treated successfully by clinical ecology practices.

HUMAN ECOLOGY ACTION LEAGUE
505 North Lake Shore Drive
Chicago, Ill. 60611

This is one of the patient groups that credits clinical ecology with the renewed health and well-being of its members. It has local chapters in 16 cities; information about these is available through this central office.

INSTITUTE FOR RESEARCH OF RHEUMATIC DISEASES
Box 955
Ansonia Station
New York, N.Y. 10023
(212) 595-1368

This group, which has two local state affiliates, has as members people who are interested in the causes and cures of the various rheumatic diseases, and the institute's aim is to further knowledge in this area.

IRRD arranges and directs seminars and conferences that are open to the public. It also publishes a quarterly newsletter, which emphasizes nutrition, and a holistic health cookbook.

LUPUS ERYTHEMATOSUS FOUNDATION, INC.
Suite 1402
95 Madison Avenue
New York, N.Y. 10016
(212) 685-4118
Director: Susan Golik

This is a local group, affiliated with the Lupus Foundation of America. Its goals are to find the cause of lupus, to improve treatment of patients, and to support research toward a cure.

The foundation provides services to patients and their families; there is a social worker on staff, and support programs are arranged. The group also distributes literature, holds meetings with guest speakers, and disseminates information to both the public and patients/families.

Membership is currently about 1200; dues are nominal.

LUPUS FOUNDATION OF AMERICA, INC.
11921 A Olive Boulevard
St. Louis, Mo. 63141
(314) 872-9036
Staff Vice President: Roger Sturdevant

This national organization has 22,000 members and 205 local chapters and groups. Mr. Sturdevant, the Staff Vice President, describes it as "a patient-oriented national voluntary health organization dedicated to informing the public about systemic lupus erythematosus; to supplying patient education and service; and to funding lupus research to find the cause and cure of the disease."

The foundation focuses on giving educational and psychological support to patients and their families. There is a nominal yearly membership fee, paid through the local chapters; information about the group is distributed free of charge to anyone who requests it.

The national foundation distributes literature about lupus, and provides counseling and referral services. It publishes a quarterly newsletter which is sent to all members through the local chapters. Funding for lupus research, in the form of grants and student summer fellowships, is also provided by the national foundation.

The local chapters offer counseling and referral services, provide physician referral lists, distribute literature about lupus, arrange support groups for patients and/or their families, and distribute chapter newsletters.

The Lupus Foundation publishes three books (see Chapter 8, *Publications*).

NATIONAL ASSOCIATION FOR HUMAN DEVELOPMENT
1620 Eye Street, N.W. #517
Washington, D.C. 20006
(202) 331-1737
President: Jules Evan Baker, Ed.D.
Executive Vice President: Anne Radd

This national organization offers health education and employment training services for older adults. Its approach includes the use of self-help materials and public awareness activities.

The issues of arthritis and rheumatic diseases are dealt with in medical workshops and publications. In addition to providing health education to older adults, NAHD also offers training sessions for those serving the elderly; for this there is a multidisciplinary faculty which includes medical practitioners, educators, and exercise physiologists.

The association provides an order form for its publications, among which are booklets on health and exercises.

NATIONAL ASSOCIATION OF THE PHYSICALLY HANDICAPPED
76 Elm Street
London, Ohio
Administrative Assistant: Helen Lee Roudebash

This non-profit organization has no services and no paid staff. Its purpose is to promote the needs of the handicapped. Membership, which costs $6 yearly, is open to both the handicapped and the non-handicapped; the only requirements are that the member be 16 or older, and a resident or citizen of the continental United States.

Among its activities are efforts to improve conditions for the handicapped in such areas as employment, housing, and transportation, both by legislative and other means. The movement for barrier-free design is a large part of the work of this group.

Recreational and social activities are organized predominantly on the local chapter level. The national office publishes a newsletter which is distributed free of charge to members; it is available to non-members on a subscription basis.

The literature from the national office stresses that it is not a resource center for information, but "a group of people supporting legislation to benefit the handicapped, and trying to make the public aware of the needs of the physically handicapped."

NATIONAL EASTER SEAL SOCIETY
2023 West Ogden Avenue
Chicago, Ill. 60612
(312) 243-8400
Executive Director: John Garrison

This national organization has a four-fold purpose: rehabilitation, advocacy, public health education, and research. In the area of rehabilitation, more than 820 state and local affiliates operate nearly 2,000 facilities and programs across the country. Among the services offered by these groups are physical and occupational therapy, vocational training, counseling, and physical and vocational evaluation.

In its role as an advocate of the handicapped, the society works with government at all levels to promote the rights of the disabled. It also supports educational programs for parents of the disabled and for self-help groups, as part of an effort to eliminate environmental and attitudinal barriers to the handicapped. The society also funds research at various institutions; these projects are focused on disabling diseases.

Fees are established for membership in the society, but no one is denied access to a service because of inability to pay.

SOCIETY FOR THE ADVANCEMENT OF TRAVEL FOR THE HANDICAPPED
26 Court Street, Suite 110
Brooklyn, N.Y. 11242
(212) 858-5483
Administration Secretary: Micki Eichler

This is a national, non-profit educational forum whose purpose is to exchange knowledge and gain new skills related to facilitating travel for the handicapped. The group publishes a newsletter, distributed to members only.

WESTERN NEW YORK ALLERGY AND ECOLOGY ASSOCIATION
1412 Colvin Boulevard
Buffalo, N.Y. 14223

This is a patients' group; its members are individuals whose illness has been relieved by clinical ecology methods.

8

PUBLICATIONS

The entries in this chapter represent a wide range of material—books, pamphlets, magazines, newsletters, and other publications that relate to the rheumatic diseases. Included also are some general publications that from time to time print articles relating directly to the treatment and/or causes of rheumatic diseases. In all, the following material provides an interesting overview of the wide diversity of attitudes and approaches to the topic.

In most cases the information in this chapter was provided by the resources themselves; some resources that did not respond to our requests for information are included because we feel they offer helpful information.

MAGAZINES AND NEWSLETTERS

ACCENT ON LIVING
  P. O.Box 700
  Bloomington, Ill. 61701
  (309) 378-2961
  Raymond C. Cheever, Editor

  Quarterly; available by subscription only ($5/year)

This publication is aimed at individuals with mobility problems. It communicates information about new products and has "how-to" hints to help the readers become more active in their daily lives.

THE AMERICAN CHIROPRACTOR
3401 Lake Avenue
Ft. Wayne, Ind. 46805
(800) 348-0757
Susan L. Bunnell, Managing Editor

Monthly; available by subscription only ($18/year)

This magazine is aimed at chiropractice professionals. It contains information about the chiropractice approach to medicine in general, and on occasion carries articles about rheumatic diseases.

AMERICAN JOURNAL OF ACUPUNCTURE
1400 Lost Acre Drive
Felton, Calif. 95018
John W. Nawratie, Editor

Quarterly; subscription is $55/year

This journal reports on advances in acupuncture, application of the technique, and other related issues.

AMERICAN JOURNAL OF CLINICAL NUTRITION
American Society for Clinical Nutrition
9650 Rockville Pike
Bethesda, Md. 20814
Dr. Albert I. Mendeloff, Editor

Monthly; $25 to members of ASCN (p. 124), $45 to non-members

Dr. Mendeloff describes this publication as "a journal reporting the practical application of our world-wide knowledge of nutrition." Articles relating directly to rheumatic diseases appear occasionally.

JOURNAL OF THE AMERICAN OSTEOPATHIC ASSOCIATION
American Osteopathic Association
212 East Ohio Street
Chicago, Ill. 60611
(213) 280-5800
George W. Northup, D.O., Editor

Monthly; available by subscription only ($10/year)

This journal, put out by AOA (p. 123), treats its subject matter from the point of view of osteopathic medicine. Accordingly, any information about arthritis will have that approach to the treatment and care of arthritis patients. Articles on the subject appear when available.

AMERICAN JOURNAL OF PHYSICAL MEDICINE
P.O. Box 617
Downtown Station,
Phoenix, Ariz. 85001
Dr. H.D. Bouman, Editor

Bi-monthly; available in some libraries, or by subscription ($20/year personal subscription, $35/year institutional; single issues, $8)

The journal is intended for people who are interested in physical medicine and rehabilitation, whether or not it is their profession.

Original articles dealing with research and clinical applications of research about arthritis appear occasionally.

AMERICAN MEDICAL NEWS
American Medical Association
535 North Dearborn Street
Chicago, Illinois 60610
(312) 751-6079

Weekly; available by subscription ($20/year)

This is the newsletter of the AMA (p. 122), which also publishes the *Journal of the AMA* (Dr. William R. Barclay, Editor), also a weekly.

ARTHRITIS NEWS TODAY
P.O. Box 730
Yorba Linda, Calif. 92686

Monthly; available by subscription only ($9/year)

This is a newsletter prepared by the Arthritis Patients Association (p. 128), and deals with the use of nutritional therapy and natural physiotherapy in the treatment of arthritis.

ASSOCIATION FOR THE CARE OF CHILDREN'S HEALTH JOURNAL AND NEWSLETTER
3615 Wisconsin Avenue
Washington, D.C. 20016
(202) 244-1801

ACCH (p. 128) publishes a quarterly journal and a bi-monthly newsletter, both of which are distributed to members as one of the services covered by their membership fees.

FAMILY HEALTH
149 Fifth Avenue
New York, N.Y. 10010
(212) 598-0800
Dalma Heyn, Editor

Monthly; available in some libraries and by subscription ($18/year; single issues, $1.50)

The magazine's articles focus on innovative approaches to diet, fitness, exercise, and nutrition, and on advances in preventive medicine and health care. The "Breakthroughs" column has items about new treatments, techniques, etc.

Family Health does not carry articles about arthritis on a regular basis, but rather when there is important and/or new information to report.

HANDY-CAP HORIZONS
Handy-Cap Horizons
3250 East Loretta Drive
Indianapolis, Ind. 46222
(317) 784-5777
Dorothy S. Axsom, Editor

This is the newsletter of Handy-Cap Horizons (p. 149), a non-profit travel club. It is sent to all members of the group; anyone at all can be a member, and dues run from $10 up, depending upon category of membership.

This publication carries information about the group itself, tours arranged by the group, new products for the handicapped, advances in research on different diseases and conditions, and inspirational notes and messages.

HEALTH CARE NEWS
5440 Cass, #211
Detroit, Michigan, 48202
(313) 831-3323
Woody Miller, Editor

Weekly; available through health professionals, in some
libraries, and by subscription ($11/year)

This newsletter is aimed at health care professionals, and reports new developments in treatment. It does not cover arthritis on a regular basis, but rather when there is new information to report.

HERALD OF HOLISTIC HEALTH
American Holistic Health Science Association
Suite 208
1766 Cumberland Green
St. Charles, Ill. 60174
(312) 377-1929

Quarterly; available by subscription only ($12/year)

This newsletter, put out by AHHSA (p. 122), contains reprints of articles from other newsletters and magazines (some in condensed form), reports pertinent to holistic health care, news items, events of different health care groups, and book reviews of appropriate titles.

Information about arthritis and its treatment is reported when available.

JOURNAL OF HOLISTIC MEDICINE
Human Sciences Press
72 Fifth Avenue
New York, N.Y. 10011
(212) 243-6000

Elmer M. Cranton, M.D., Editor
P. O. Box 44
Trout Dale, Va. 24378

Bi-annual; available in some libraries and by subscription
($45 in the U.S., $48 in Canada, $51 in foreign countries)

This is the official journal of the American Holistic Medicine Association and is aimed at holistic health professionals. The journal publishes articles concerning various disciplines of holistic care, including nutrition, physical exercise, acupuncture, environmental medicine, behavioral therapies, and voluntary self-regulation.

Special emphasis is given to less well-known and non-traditional methods of diagnosis and treatment that have been proven safe and effective.

LUPUS ERYTHEMATOSUS FOUNDATION, INC.
NEWSLETTERS
Suite 1402
95 Madison Avenue
New York, N.Y. 10016
(212) 685-4118

The SLE Foundation (p. 130) is an affiliate of the Lupus Foundation of America (p. 130). It publishes its own newsletters throughout the year, which are distributed free to members. These are aimed at patients and the general public. The foundation also publishes some compilations of reprint articles relating to lupus. These are:

COPING WITH DEPRESSION IN A CHRONIC ILLNESS
LUPUS AND YOU: A GUIDE FOR PATIENTS
LUPUS ERYTHEMATOSUS: A HANDBOOK FOR PHYSICIANS, PATIENTS, AND THEIR FAMILIES
LUPUS ERYTHEMATOSUS: VOLUMES 1, 2, 3 (This set is published by the Atlanta chapter of the Lupus Foundation, but is distributed by the New York chapter as well.)

MEDICAL ABSTRACTS NEWSLETTERS
586 Teaneck Road
Teaneck, N.J. 07666
Toni Goldfarb, Editor

Monthly; available by subscription only ($18/year or $10 for a six-month trial subscription)

This newsletter is exactly what its title says, a compilation of abstracts from other medical publications. Each is attributed to its original source, thereby enabling the reader to find the complete report in its original journal. The newsletter has an advisory board of nine doctors, each a specialist in a different field. The publication does not take any point of view, nor does it provide medical advice.

Any specific mention of rheumatic diseases depends on such mention in other medical journals.

MEDICAL SELF CARE
P.O. Box 718
Inverness, Calif. 94937
Dr. Tom Ferguson, Editor

Quarterly; available on some newsstands, in some libraries, and by subscription ($15/year; single issues, $4).

This magazine is aimed at health consumer activists, educators, and practitioners.

NATIONAL ARTHRITIS NEWS
Arthritis Foundation
1314 Spring Street
Atlanta, Ga. 30309
(404) 872-7100

The Arthritis Foundation (p. 127) has many publications. Some are aimed at the general public, others are for professionals who treat and deal with arthritis and rheumatic diseases.

NAN (National Arthritis News) is a quarterly membership publication that reports on the various activities of member groups around the country.

There is a series of booklets on medications, one on forms of arthritis, and another on living with arthritis. These are usually furnished free of charge to people who request them.

The foundation also publishes a primer on arthritis, a bulletin, and a journal for physicians and researchers.

NATIONAL ASSOCIATION OF THE PHYSICALLY HANDICAPPED
    76 Elm Street
    London, Ohio 43140

NAPH (p. 131) publishes a quarterly newsletter that discusses various aspects of rehabilitation, information about new self-help aids, events pertaining to the handicapped, legislation, etc. It is free with membership in the organization, or can be obtained by subscription ($3/year).

NATURAL HEALTH AND FITNESS BULLETIN
    CN 5245
    Princeton, N.J. 08540
    (609) 924-9320
    Carlson Wade, Editor

    Monthly; available by subscription only ($28/year)

This bulletin is aimed at the general consumer. It advocates a more natural method of treatment with minimal drug use. Information pertinent to rheumatic diseases is published when available.

ORTHOPOD
    American Osteopathic Academy of Orthopedics
    1217 Salem Avenue
    Dayton, Ohio 45406
    (513) 274-7151
    Daniel Morrison, D.O., Editor

    Published two or three times yearly; available in some
    libraries, and by subscription (rates upon request)

This magazine is aimed at osteopathic orthopedic surgeons. Its concern with arthritis is strictly limited to "the surgical approach to advanced arthritis in various areas." Articles pertaining to rheumatic diseases are printed when they are available.

PREVENTION Magazine
    33 East Minor Street
    Emmaus, Pa. 18049
    Robert Rodale, Editor

    Monthly; available on newsstands, in libraries, and by
    subscription

This magazine was one of the first in the country to advocate natural remedies for illness. Vitamins and minerals are discussed in great depth; over the course of a year or two nearly every nutritional supplement is explained, with case studies often included. The magazine also prints recipes for healthful foods. There is a reader's information column, in which anecdotes and experiences related to nutrition are shared.

Articles concerning the various forms of arthritis are published from time to time.

PROGRAMS FOR THE HANDICAPPED
Clearinghouse on the Handicapped
Office of Special Education and
   Rehabilitative Services
U.S. Department of Education
Room 3119 Switzer Building
Washington, D.C. 20202
(202) 245-0080

Clearinghouse on the Handicapped (p. 148) publishes some useful guides. Among them is the bi-monthly publication *Programs for the Handicapped*, which focuses on federal activities that benefit the handicapped. It serves the interest of professionals, administrators, and others concerned with the needs of the disabled.

SATH NEWSLETTER
Society for the Advancement of Travel for the Handicapped
26 Court Street
Brooklyn, N.Y. 11242
(212) 858-5483

Bi-monthly; available with membership only

This newsletter is aimed at the travel industry as well as the handicapped, and those interested in travel for the handicapped. It includes a column that notes other publications of interest, articles about special events for the handicapped, information about SATH events, and even information about accommodations for the handicapped at different companies.

SOCIETY FOR CLINICAL ECOLOGY NEWSLETTER
Suite 490
2005 Franklin Street
Denver, Colo. 80205
(303) 622-9755

The Society for Clinical Ecology (p. 127) publishes a newsletter on a quarterly basis. Non-members may subscribe to it, at a cost of $16/year. Checks should be made payable to the Society for Clinical Ecology Newsletter, and orders sent to: X-Press! Publishing, Box U, North Bend, Wash. 98045.

There is a list of other publications, mainly books, about clinical ecology and/or written by clinical ecologists. This publications list can be obtained from Dickey Enterprises, 635 Gregory Road, Ft. Collins, Colo. 80524; (303) 482-6001. The books on the list vary from those written for the professional to those intended for the general public.

WESTERN JOURNAL OF MEDICINE
44 Gough Street
San Francisco, Calif. 94103
Malcolm S. J. Watts, M.D., Editor

Monthly; available by prepaid subscription ($10/year; single issues, $2.50 prepaid)

This journal is intended for medical professionals. It reports on advances in medicine and research findings. The coverage of arthritis and other rheumatic diseases takes the form of occasional updates on proven treatments.

BOOKS AND PAMPHLETS

ACCESS AIRPORTS
Consumer Information Center
Department A
Pueblo, Colo. 81009

ACCESS AIRPORTS details the airports in the United States and their accessibility for the handicapped. It is free.

The booklet is published by a government agency called Consumer Information Center. Most material from this agency is free, or available at a nominal fee. Write and request to be put on the mailing list for catalogs.

ACTIVITIES FOR CHILDREN WITH SPECIAL NEEDS
Association for the Care of Children's Health
3615 Wisconsin Avenue
Washington, D.C. 200165
(202) 244-1801

This book costs $3 for non-members.

A DOCTOR DISCUSSES ARTHRITIS, RHEUMATISM, AND GOUT
Robert E. Dunbar with Harold F. Seegall, M.D.
Published by Budlong Press
Distributed by Milex Products, 5915 Northwest Highway, Chicago, Ill. 60631

This book is consistent with conventional medical thinking about these diseases. It contains thorough discussions of drug therapy, surgery, and physiotherapy. Exercises are illustrated, and sources for self-help devices are included.

AIR TRAVEL FOR THE HANDICAPPED
TWA Sales Department
2 Penn Plaza
New York, N.Y. 10010

This pamphlet, distributed free of charge, may be obtained by writing to any TWA sales office throughout the United States, or by visiting any TWA travel store.

The information contained in the pamphlet concerns air travel for people with limited mobility. Hints about making your reservation, arrival at the airport, what the airline personnel can and cannot do, and other such areas of interest make this a valuable guide.

A LEGAL MANUAL FOR LUPUS PATIENTS
Lupus Foundation of America, Inc.
11921 A Olive Boulevard
St. Louis, Mo. 63141
(314) 872-9036
Elizabeth J. Jameson and Susan L. Bloom (Attorneys) and
Ronald Carr, M.D., Authors

This is a handbook on Social Security disability and patients' rights. It costs $5 plus $1 for postage and handling; checks should be made out to the Lupus Foundation of America, Inc.

AMERICAN OCCUPATIONAL THERAPY ASSOCIATION
INFORMATION PACKETS
1383 Piccard Drive
Rockville, Md. 20815
(301) 948-9626

AOTA publishes a series of packets that cover various aspects of occupational therapy practice and contain current reference material. Each packet includes the names of personnel; specific questions on the various topics may be addressed to these individuals. The series is called the *Practice Division Information Packets.* There are packets about adapted clothing, adapted equipment, and arthritis. AOTA members receive the first packet free, with subsequent packets costing $5 each. Non-members may order the packets at $6.50 each.

A Workbook for Consumers with Rheumatoid Arthritis—Joint Protection Principles for Rheumatoid Arthritis is an illustrated workbook for patients, intended to be used with the assistance of an occupational therapist. The cost is $3 each (1–40 copies, or $2.50 each for 41 copies or more) for members; $4.50 each for non-members ($4 each for 41 copies or more).

ARTHRITIS AND HOW TO DEAL WITH IT
Merck, Sharp, and Dohme
Health Information Services
P.O. Box 1486
North Wales, Pa. 19454
Vera Belsky, Editorial Director

This is a very basic information pamphlet. It describes the major forms of arthritis, stressing the importance of medical treatment. It is an Arthritis Foundation (p. 127) publication, distributed by the pharmaceutical company Merck, Sharp, and Dohme. Individual copies are free upon request; bulk orders costs $3 for 25 copies.

ARTHRITIS AND RHEUMATISM
Arthritis Foundation
American Rheumatism Association Section
1314 Spring Street
Atlanta, Ga. 30309
(404) 872-7100, ext. 209
Dr. J. Claude Bennett, Editor

This book deals specifically with the issues of rheumatic diseases, their treatment, causes, and research into possible cures. It is published by the Arthritis Foundation (p. 127).

ARTHRITIS INFORMATION CLEARINGHOUSE CATALOG
P.O. Box 9782
Arlington, Va. 22209

This clearinghouse (p. 147) prints a catalog of its publications and will send it upon request. The material listed in the catalog includes bibliographies, catalogs, and reference sheets. In addition, an individualized data base bibliography on topics of special interest may be obtained upon request.

ARTHRITIS REMEDIES FROM AROUND THE WORLD
Health-Wealth Publishers
P.O. Box 91
Niagara Falls, N.Y. 14305

This softcover booklet discusses both conventional treatments used by allopathic doctors and alternative, controversial remedies. It costs $4.95.

ARTHRITIS: THE FACTS
P.O. Box 700
Bloomington, Ill. 61701
(309) 378-2961
Raymond C. Cheever, Editor

Published by *Accent on Living*, this book costs $5.95 plus 65¢ postage.

BECKY'S STORY
Association for the Care of Children's Health
3615 Wisconsin Avenue
Washington, D.C. 20016
(202) 244-1801

This is a book for siblings of hospitalized children. Non-members may buy the book for $3.

COPING WITH CHRONIC PAIN
Mensana Clinic
1718 Greenspring Valley Road
Stevenson, Md. 21153
(301) 652-2403
N. Hendler, M.D., and J. Alsofrom Fenton, Editors

This book is written for patients and their families in non-technical, clear terminology. $10 plus $1 postage and handling.

DIAGNOSIS AND NONSURGICAL MANAGEMENT OF CHRONIC PAIN
Mensana Clinic
1718 Greenspring Valley Road
Stevenson, Md. 21153
(301) 652-2403
N. Hendler, M.D., Editor

This is a comprehensive textbook; it provides a multidisciplinary approach. It costs $34 plus $1 postage and handling.

DIAGNOSIS AND TREATMENT OF CHRONIC PAIN
Mensana Clinic
1718 Greenspring Valley Road
Stevenson, Md. 21153
(301) 652-2403
N. Hendler, M.D., D. Long, M.D., T. Wise, M.D., Editors

This is a clinician-oriented reference work. It discusses every aspect of problems with chronic pain. $22.50 plus $1 postage and handling.

DIRECTORY OF INFORMATION AND REFERRAL SERVICES
Alliance of Information and Referral Systems
1100 West 452nd Street
Indianapolis, Ind. 46208
(317) 923-8727
Director: Dr. Karen S. Haynes

AIRS has just published the *Directory of Information and Referral Services.* Although it does not relate to the rheumatic diseases directly, the information in this volume may prove useful to those who want or need to know where to turn for referrals related to their condition or circumstances. The directory costs $15 for members of the alliance, $17 for non-members.

GOING PLACES IN YOUR OWN VEHICLE
P.O. Box 700
Bloomington, Ill. 61701
(309) 378-2961
Raymond C. Cheever, Editor

This book, published by *Accent on Living*, costs $6.50 plus 65¢ postage.

GUIDELINES FOR ADOLESCENT UNITS
Association for the Care of Children's Health
3615 Wisconsin Avenue
Washington, D.C. 20016
(202) 244-1801

This book, published by ACCH (p. 128), outlines the philosophy and standards for adolescent units in hospitals: $3 for non-members.

HIGHWAY REST AREA FACILITIES DESIGNED FOR HANDICAPPED TRAVELLERS
President's Committee on Employment of the Handicapped
Washington, D.C.
(202) 653-5044
Director: Bernard Posner

This booklet lists, on a state-by-state basis, the facilities at the different highway rest areas that are designed to be accessible to the handicapped.

The booklet is put out by the President's Committee on Employment of the Handicapped, which publishes material on employment, clothing for the handicapped, independent living ideas, and other areas of interest for disabled people.

All the publications from this office are free of charge. A list of all titles is available upon request.

HOPE FOR THE ARTHRITIC
John Lust, N.D.
25 Dewart Road
Greenwich, Conn. 06803

This publication is updated bi-annually. It is available from the author/publisher, and in some libraries. It advocates a drugless treatment, using natural methods including nutrition, hydrotherapy, and botanical medications. The cost is $2.95 per copy.

IDEAS FOR MAKING YOUR HOME ACCESSIBLE
P.O. Box 700
Bloomington, Ill. 61701
(309) 378-2961

This book is published by *Accent on Living*, and costs $6.50 plus 65¢ for postage.

LUPUS ERYTHEMATOSUS: A HANDBOOK FOR PHYSICIANS, PATIENTS, AND THEIR FAMILIES
Lupus Foundation of America, Inc.
11921 A Olive Boulevard
St. Louis, Mo. 63141
(314) 872-9036

Copies of this pamphlet may be bought for $1 each. Checks should be made payable to the Lupus Foundation of America, Inc.

LUPUS, HOPE THROUGH UNDERSTANDING
Lupus Foundation of America, Inc.
11921 A Olive Boulevard
St. Louis, Mo. 63141
(314) 872-9036
Henrietta Aladjem, Author (1982)

This book costs $7 plus $1 for postage and handling. Checks should be made payable to the Lupus Foundation of America, Inc.

NATIONAL ASSOCIATION FOR HUMAN DEVELOPMENT DIGEST
1620 Eye Street, N.W. #517
Washington, D.C. 20006
(202) 331-1737

This publication, put out quarterly by NAHD (p. 130), is devoted to health information appropriate for older adults (coping with chronic diseases, exercise and diet for good health, etc.).

NATIONAL EASTER SEAL SOCIETY CATALOG
2023 West Ogden Avenue
Chicago, Ill. 60612
(312) 243-8400

This national foundation (p. 131) has prepared a catalog of its publications. The catalog is revised annually. Among the publications are those appropriate for health professionals, people with disabilities, and families of the disabled. Some of the society's pamphlets are available in Spanish. There are bibliographies available, and many of the items have lower rates when bought in quantity.

NATIONAL HOMECARING COUNCIL CATALOG
235 Park Avenue South
New York, N.Y. 10003
(212) 674-4990

NHC (p. 126), which has as its purpose the establishment and maintenance of standards for home health care, publishes books, pamphlets, papers, and other materials that apply to the organization's function. A (1982–1983) catalog of publications and audiovisual aids is available. NHC literature includes material for the consumer and for professionals who specialize in the field of chronic illnesses.

NEW LIFE, OLD HANDS
Dow Corning Corporation
Department 5107
Midland, Mich. 48640

This booklet was prepared in cooperation with the Arthritis Foundation (p. 127). It discusses the reconstruction of deformed, diseased, or destroyed joints of the hand, wrist, elbow, and foot by surgery, using flexible implants.

The booklet is available free of charge upon written request (a postcard will suffice).

RESOURCE GUIDE: EMPLOYMENT OF THE HANDICAPPED
(1982)
Clearinghouse on the Handicapped
Office of Special Education and Rehabilitative Services
U.S. Department of Education
Room 3119 Switzer Building
Washington, D.C. 20202
(202) 245-0080

Geared toward professionals, this book describes the type of employment assistance that is available from the government and from private, national organizations. It is one of several Clearinghouse (p. 148) publications.

RESOURCE GUIDE: REHABILITATION ENGINEERING AND PRODUCT INFORMATION (1980)
Clearinghouse on the Handicapped
Office of Special Education and Rehabilitative Services
U.S. Department of Education
Room 3119 Switzer Building
Washington, D.C. 20202
(202) 245-0080

This book offers information about technological research and available products. It is one of several Clearinghouse (p. 148) publications.

WHEELCHAIRS AND ACCESSORIES
P.O. Box 700
Bloomington, Ill. 61701
(309) 378-2961
Raymond C. Cheever, Editor

Published by *Accent on Living*, this book costs $7.50 plus 65¢ postage.

9

SERVICES

The information in this chapter pertains to various services available to patients with rheumatic disease. Some of these are information services, others are sources of self-help aids and products. Hotlines for information, guidance and counseling services, and travel services are part of the wide range of facilities that exist to help patients and/or their families.

ARTHRITIS INFORMATION CLEARINGHOUSE
P.O. Box 9782
Arlington, Va. 22209
(703) 558-8250

This clearinghouse is a division of the National Institute of Arthritis, Diabetes, and Digestive and Kidney Diseases (p. 126). The purpose of this section is to identify, collect, process, and make available information about the various educational materials concerned with the rheumatic diseases.

Direct aid to patients and/or their families is not part of the function of the clearinghouse; rather, the work done here is aimed at professionals who need or want more information about the various conditions. For example, a doctor who wants to know what literature is available concerning the use of a particular medication can call the "Searchline" (at the same phone number listed above) and ask. The AIC staff will then compile the information requested.

The Clearinghouse deals with printed matter, audiovisual materials, and from these prepares bibliographies, reference sheets, catalogs (p. 142), guides, and reports. Inclusion of an item in an AIC-prepared listing is not a recommendation or endorsement by AIC or NIADDK. All AIC services are free of charge.

CLEARINGHOUSE ON THE HANDICAPPED
Office of Special Education and Rehabilitative Services
Department of Education
Switzer Building, Room 3119
Washington, D.C. 20202
(202) 245-0080
Director: Helga Roth, Ph.D.

The services of this clearinghouse are available to anyone. Inquiries may be made by phone call, letter, or personal visit. The purpose of this group is to make the exchange of information relating to disabilities easier for those who are disabled and for the providers of services to the disabled.

Although the clearinghouse has information from many different sources, its special strength lies in the areas of federal funding for programs serving disabled people, federal legislation affecting the handicapped, and federal programs benefiting people with handicapping conditions.

When it receives inquiries regarding actual services, the Clearinghouse will refer the request to resources as close, geographically, to the correspondent as possible.

EVERGREEN TRAVEL SERVICE, INC.
19505 "L" 44th Avenue, West
Lynnwood, Wash. 98036
(206) 776-1184
Director: Betty J. Hoffman

This travel service specializes in tours for handicapped clients. It has been in service for 25 years, during which time its director, Betty Hoffman, has led tours to every inhabited continent.

Each tour is escorted by Mrs. Hoffman and her son; the tour group is composed of people with the same handicap. Among the special tours arranged and escorted by the Hoffmans were visits to a clinic in Romania that specializes in the treatment of arthritis (Dr. Aslan), and a clinic in Italy that uses the same methods.

FLYING WHEELS TRAVEL
Box 382
Owatonna, Minn. 55060
(800) 533-0363
Vice President: Barbara Jacobson
Manager: Sharon Schleich

Flying Wheels arranges group and individual travel plans for the physically handicapped. Group tours are limited to 25 people, including the Flying Wheels escort. Travelers require a companion only if they are unable to dress and care for themselves. In those cases, an able-bodied companion must come along. A participant can request that Flying Wheels provide one, or may bring a campanion of his or her choice.

SERVICES   149

The Flying Wheels escort is trained in the medical field in order to assist with any daily routines (medications, etc.) that may be required.
The tours have included travel through Europe and the United States, both by air and by sea. Cruises to nearby resort areas are also among the travel plans arranges by Flying Wheels. Individual trips can be handled by this service; it has the experience to incorporate the special needs of the handicapped into travel plans.
A fee of $2 will cover the cost of newsletters and mailings from Flying Wheels.

HANDI-RAMP, INC.
1414 Armour Boulevard
Mundelein, Ill. 60060
This company manufactures and distributes Handi-Ramp, a fold-away ramp designed primarily for wheelchair users. It can be used with vehicles, or where there is a high curb, or a rise to a doorway. The advantage of the fold-away ramp is that it is portable.

HANDY-CAP HORIZONS
3250 East Loretta Drive
Indianapolis, Ind. 46222
(317) 784-5777
President: Dorothy S. Axsom
This is a non-profit travel club; its purpose and goal is to get "special people out of homes into the world through vacation, education, training, and work toward legislation for more 'live-able' lives."
There are membership dues of $10/year and up, which entitle the member to a subscription to *Handy-Cap Horizons* (the quarterly newsletter, p. 135), all membership mailings, and eligibility for tours and activities. The membership is national and is open to anyone, regardless of physical condition. The tours are strictly limited to members and are usually at a discounted price because of the group's non-profit status.
One stipulation regarding the tours is that if a member is not completely capable physically, he or she must have a helper or companion. The office maintains files of members who are interested in accompanying handicapped members, who pay part of the companion's expenses.

INFORMATION CENTER FOR INDIVIDUALS WITH
    DISABILITIES
Suite 330
20 Park Plaza
Boston, Mass. 02116
(617) 727-5540
(800) 462-5015, within Massachusetts
(617) 727-5236, for the hearing impaired
Director: Sandra Bouzoukis
This is a national group that provides information and referrals for people with disabilities, agencies that help people with disabilities, and/or families and friends of the disabled.

All information and referrals are free of charge. ICID deals with such topics as accessibility, housing, law, finance, equipment, education, human relations, recreation, travel, transportation, and employment. Inquiries may be made by phone, in writing, or through a personal visit.

JUST ONE BREAK
373 Park Avenue South
New York, N.Y. 10016
(212) 725-2500
Director: Paul Hearne

This service is a local one, available to adults at no charge. Its main purpose is "job placement and supportive services for the physically and mentally disabled."

To fulfill its stated goal, Just One Break provides a full range of services. The job placement service is well-known in the New York metropolitan area, and employers from all over the area list opportunities with JOB. The supportive services are comprehensive. The organization will help a client evaluate his or her vocational abilities and interests. Research into the employment market is conducted; so is counseling. JOB also offers technical assistance to prepare a client for a job or to help that person keep a job.

MADDAK, INC.
Pequannock, N.J. 07440
(201) 694-0500
Marketing Manager: Steven Levine

This company manufactures and distributes self-help aids and homecare products. These aids are available for children as well as adults.

The catalog, which is free upon written request (a postcard will suffice), contains a full complement of implements that will make daily chores easier for anyone who is disabled by a rheumatic disease. In addition to canes, walkers, wheelchairs, and accessories, Maddak sells a wide variety of hand exercisers (including the Hand Gym® exercise unit), equipment for heat and cold therapy, items to make holding things easier, dressing aids, grooming and eating aids, and splints. The range of household aids is also comprehensive.

MOBILITY TOURS
Suite 1110
26 Court Street
Brooklyn, N.Y. 11242
(212) 858-6021
(212) 625-4744, for the hearing impaired
Director: Ronni Trabman
Assistant: Melanie S. Mandel

Mobility Tours arranges group tours for disabled people. The tours range from one-day excursions to cruises, with all variations between the two. Some of the tours travel by motorcoach, and these vehicles are equipped to handle wheelchairs and special seating needs. The tours are planned with the special needs of the handicapped taken into consideration.

Mobility Tours has a program called Mobility Sports, which arranges sports-oriented outings or trips. Each has a different sport or activity as its focus (among the choices are photography and nature walks, fishing, and weekend camping). Participation depends on the individual's capabilities.

Another service of Mobility Tours is the rental of specially equipped mini-vans, separate from arranged tours. These vans have hydraulic lifts to accommodate wheelchairs as well as various luxury features to make a journey more comfortable.

NATIONAL HOMECARING COUNCIL
235 Park Avenue South
New York, N.Y. 10003
(212) 674-4990

Among the functions of this organization (p. 126) is the accreditation of homecaring agencies throughout the country. NHC will provide a list of accredited agencies in each state upon request. (See also p. 145, for publications.)

NATIONAL INSTITUTE FOR REHABILITATION
  ENGINEERING
97 Decker Road
Butler, N.J. 07405
(201) 838-2500
(201) 838-2578, for the hearing impaired
Technical Director: Donald Selwyn

This national organization was founded to help the handicapped through the use of modern technology. Medical professionals and engineers work together to design equipment and technological aids that will help severely handicapped people. NIRE has already devised special wheelchairs, adapted office machines, self-help aids, dressing and personal care aids, and special clothing that are designed to make occupational and daily tasks easier for the individual, thereby increasing independence.

NIRE works on individual cases, after all other means of rehabilitation have been investigated by the client. Initial consultations on the problem are free of charge and carry no obligation. Once the engineers and medical professionals have analyzed the problem to be solved and have devised a solution, the client has the opportunity to discuss the plan with the staff at NIRE; fees for the service/aids are discussed at that time. Fees for most services are on a sliding scale basis, related to the client's income and means.

The cost of some of the aids and services may be covered by some insurance policies; wheelchairs, for example, usually are covered. Clients may be of any age; NIRE's focus is on the technological aspects of the problem to be solved.

J.A. PRESTON CORPORATION
60 Page Road
Clifton, N.J. 07012
(800) 631-7277
(201) 777-2700

This company manufactures and distributes equipment and aids for use by arthritics and anyone with disabilities. The aids and equipment are available for children as well as adults.

A catalog will be sent free of charge upon request. It shows a full range of aids and devices that increase the independence of anyone with physical restrictions. Among the products are exercisers, dressing aids, eating aids, various splints, grooming aids, and household aids. All of these are intended to help make daily tasks easier.

RESOURCE CENTER
Hassel Library
Moss Rehabilitation Hospital
12th Street and Tabor Road
Philadelphia, Pa. 19141
(215) 329-5715

This center is a library of information on all aspects of physical disability and rehabilitation. It contains information on special programs for the disabled, services available to them, facilities, and legal rights.

The center operates a lending library, providing access to printed and audiovisual material. Free literature is available there, and it will refer inquiries to other agencies on a limited basis. One of the center's functions is the sponsorship of workshops for both the disabled and professionals who work in rehabilitative disciplines.

Rehab Line is a telephone information service that has taped information; ask for the brochure that lists the specific messages. The phone number is *(215) 329-0838;* "*Rehab Line*" is in operation Monday through Friday, from 9 a.m. to 5 p.m., except on major holidays.

SOUTHERN PROSTHETIC SUPPLY COMPANY
947 Juniper Street, N.E.
Atlanta, Ga. 30309
(404) 872-1777

This company distributes orthotic materials and other physical aids useful to people with disabilities. A catalog of products is available upon request.

TEL-MED CORPORATION
P.O. Box 22700
Cooley Drive
Colton, Calif.
(714) 825-7000

This company supplies free health information. It has a network of telephone numbers throughout the United States that the user can call to hear individual tape-recorded messages. Each pertains to a different health topic: diseases, conditions, rehabilitation information, etc.

To obtain the most current listing of phone numbers, either write or call Tel-Med at the central office (above). At the same time, request the current listing of tapes. Each has a number and title. When you call your local number, tell the Tel-Med operator which tape you want to hear, using both the number and title. Also, ask the operator to send you the listing of locally prepared tapes; some of the branch offices have prepared additional recordings which are not part of the national listing. There are tapes on gout, arthritis and rheumatism, rheumatoid arthritis, and bursitis.

TRAVEL INFORMATION CENTER
Moss Rehabilitation Hospital
12th Street and Tabor Road
Philadelphia, Pa. 19141
(215) 329-5715

This center sends information on travel: where to visit, different ways to get there, what to see once you are there, where to stay. It is NOT a travel agency, and will not make arrangements. The staff will talk with travel agents, however, if the need arises.

An individual wishing to travel should call the center and outline which cities or countries are of interest and what his or her special interest areas are (archaeology, art, etc.). The center will then collect information about that location from its resources, and send it to the caller. This material includes such details as information about the sites themselves, how accessible they are to the disabled, and the names of other agencies, groups, or individuals who can supply more information. The caller can then contact a travel agent to arrange the trip.

TIC requests that anyone using its services report back after a trip, so that the information in the center's library can be kept up to date. All TIC services are free.

VOCATIONAL GUIDANCE AND REHABILITATION
SERVICES
2239 East 55th Street
Cleveland, Ohio 44103
(216) 431-7800
President: Theodore Fabyn

This is a private, non-profit social service agency, active in the Cleveland area only. It was established to help those people who have "barriers to employment," such as the disabled, find jobs.

VGRS offers a physical capacities evaluation series designed to determine a client's ability to perform work, endurance, handling and fingering ability, motor skills, etc. The results will help the client avoid wasting time investigating inappropriate jobs and will identify the type of work the client *can* do.

Work evaluation is a primary process in helping the client find employment. Vocational and "hands-on" testing are among the procedures used to help identify the most promising opportunity for the client.

VGRS also offers psychological and vocational testing, and vocational and educational counseling, for those clients who require any or all of those services.

The organization arranges some work programs for those clients whose skills/abilities fit; others are placed in individual jobs.

.

INDEX

Names of health professionals, hospitals, and clinics, with descriptive information about treatment approach, insurance coverage, etc., are given alphabetically in directory section, pp. 81–119. Names of professional associations, foundations, organizations, and self-help groups are given alphabetically in the directory pp. 120–32. Publications on rheumatic diseases are listed alphabetically by title pp. 133–46. An alphabetical directory of services to patients appears on pp. 147–54

BAYX HOP

F

93